A PROPER MOTHER

A PROPER MOTHER

ISOBEL SHIRLAW

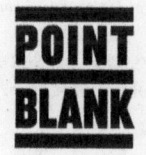

POINT BLANK

A POINT BLANK BOOK

First published in Great Britain, the Republic of Ireland and Australia by Point Blank, an imprint of Oneworld Publications, 2024

Copyright © Isobel Shirlaw, 2024

The moral right of Isobel Shirlaw to be identified as the Author of this work has been asserted by her in accordance with the Copyright, Designs and Patents Act 1988

All rights reserved
Copyright under Berne Convention
A CIP record for this title is available from the British Library

ISBN 978-0-86154-698-5
eISBN 978-0-86154-722-7

Printed and bound in Great Britain by Clays Ltd, Elcograf S.p.A.

This book is a work of fiction. Names, characters, businesses, organisations, places and events are either the product of the author's imagination or are used fictitiously. Any resemblance to actual persons, living or dead, events or locales is entirely coincidental.

Oneworld Publications
10 Bloomsbury Street
London WC1B 3SR
England

Stay up to date with the latest books, special offers, and exclusive content from Oneworld with our newsletter

Sign up on our website
oneworld-publications.com/point-blank

MIX
Paper | Supporting responsible forestry
FSC® C018072

For R, R and N

BEFORE

August 1974

On the last day of their honeymoon, they thought they'd check out Agios Ioannis. Frankie had read in the guide book that although the cove was charming, tourists hardly ever went there because, unlike most of the other beaches on the island, it was small and fairly out of the way, unless you had a car, that is. But for those who persevered, it was well worth it, apparently.

So they hired a car for the day – a rusty black Renault with no seatbelts, a broken brake light and a cardboard air-freshener that swung, suspended by a string of brown prayer beads, from the rear-view mirror, emitting such a pungent fusion of citronella and furniture polish that they almost didn't notice the crack that snaked across their horizon as they set off after breakfast before it got too hot.

Instead of turning right at the top of the main town, and down towards the harbour, they went the other way – the road climbing further and further up until they were approaching the island's summit.

Frankie checked the map in the book as they juddered along. There was a chapel up on the rocks, it said, on the site of an ancient Byzantine monastery that had burnt down over three hundred years ago, and a shrine nearby, where two children in the 1930s had reportedly witnessed a vision of the Virgin Mary. There was a taverna, too, in the village of the same name, a couple of kilometres over the headland, run by a Daphne Mandrapilias – of the famous Mandrapilias Circus family – and her husband, Vasilis.

'Daphne Mandrapilias,' Frankie said to herself, imagining the owner of such an exotic name, frowning slightly as she pictured Daphne – lithe in a sequinned bikini, swinging from a trapeze. She checked her hair in the splintered wing mirror. It had lightened in the sun and she noticed the way her olive-green and gold striped going-away dress emphasised the flecks in her hazel eyes. She sat up straighter and turned her face to one side. Although the fabric was a bit scratchy, it hung pleasingly on her collar bone, reminding her just a tiny bit, whatever Callum might have said, of that little picture of Lauren Bacall with her second husband that she'd cut out of an old bridal magazine for the hairdresser.

When the Carpenters came on, Callum winced, fiddling with the radio until the fizzing dissolved into a tinny Greek pop song that Frankie had no recollection of having heard before. But by the time it finished playing, Callum was humming along as if he'd known it all his life. He winked at her, resting a hand – hot – on her thigh. Realising he must have seen her admiring her reflection, she squinted, pretending to wipe a speck of dust from her eye.

Callum's perennial tan had darkened to such a deep nutty colour that people had been speaking Greek to him all week. She didn't need to tell him how much it suited him and had been a little irritated when he, too, had looked over to notice the group of Greek girls watching him when he came out of the sea the previous morning, his faded red shorts slung low to expose a bright white stripe across his hips. She realised, glancing over at him – one elbow resting on the window frame – that he'd been singing not just for the whole journey, but for most of the holiday.

She had been feeling queasy for several days and the air-freshener wasn't helping. Turning her face to the window, she closed her eyes and breathed in the hot dry aroma of pine and oregano as she tried to block out the smell of the car, not to mention the vision of the farm back home – sulking – in the dark and the rain, counting the hours until their return. She frowned, wondering how they were ever going to tear themselves away from this paradise the next day.

The sparse vegetation thinned out in time with the music, which grew more and more distant – like a child singing through a hurricane – until the road abandoned them altogether, leaving only a sandy track that looked as if it had been designed exclusively for donkeys. The car struggled to climb, tyres spinning in the dust. Callum swore under his breath as he tried to get it moving but it wouldn't budge. And in the end, they got out and pushed it the final few metres to the top.

Everything was greener on the other side. But as the windscreen wipers scraped away the sand, Frankie was alarmed to see that the way down was narrow and steep, with almost no verge between the wheels and the cliff face. She gripped the door handle with one hand, Callum's knee with the other, and didn't open her eyes until they reached the bottom.

They parked on a desolate patch of gorse which suggested the edge of a dune but which gave way unexpectedly, a few metres on, to a strangely lunar landscape of bright white rock, adorned with large gleaming boulders.

Callum spotted a cleft in the rock that revealed, up close, a thin ravine of sand. Someone had drilled a spindly yellow rope banister into the side of the rock to guide people down to the beach, reminding Frankie – as she clung on, awkwardly – of a loosely carpeted staircase in an old country house.

She slipped, bashing her foot against the rock, and cried out, her hand flying instinctively to her stomach. Her toe was bleeding and she felt a flash of annoyance at Callum for not waiting, envying his easy barefoot agility as he dug his heels firmly in the sand, letting himself fall, in a steady gliding tread, like a skier, before clambering over the remaining rocks without so much as a glance over his shoulder.

The rocks concealed a perfectly formed cove, the colour of honeycomb. There was no-one else there. And the sea – prickling under the stark angry sun – was as still as a lake.

She hobbled over the burning sand and crouched down at the water's edge to wash the blood off her foot. Callum came up behind her. 'Look at the colour of that water.' He grabbed her around the waist, as if to throw her in, so that she stumbled.

'Careful,' she said, too sharply.

He kissed her on the back of the neck. 'What are you waiting for?' he whispered, running one finger down her spine.

She leant back into him.

'Get your cossie on.' He waded out, snorkel dangling loosely from his slack jaw as he kicked the water behind him. 'And if you're lucky,' he shouted, 'when we get out, maybe I'll help you take it off again.'

They left the beach just after one. Although Frankie felt they ought to visit the chapel, Callum was hungry, reckoning it would take a good hour or two to climb all the way up there – with no shade, either. The sun was directly overhead now, so that as they climbed the hill to the village, it felt as though someone were pressing drawing pins into her scalp. She reached into her bag for the thermos; they'd left it in the footwell of the car all morning and the water was warm with a strong petrol aftertaste. She was unsettled by how still everything was – as if the sun – having once been humiliated by the breeze – hadn't yet decided whether to let it go.

Before

Something caught her eye on the other side of the road – a little blue and white wooden shrine, like a bird house, on stilts. Inside was a candle, two plastic lilies and a tiny metal painting propped up against the back of the wood – an ikon, she realised, peering closer – of the Madonna and child, nestling in a bed of white ribbon that cradled a pair of powder-blue knitted baby shoes.

So this was the actual place where those children had their vision, she realised, half-remembering something she'd read in the guide book, and she called out to Callum to wait, but he'd already disappeared around the corner. The chapel must have been built later. She tried to picture them – laughing – barefoot in the dust and wondered where they'd been going that day – if they'd recognised the Virgin – whether she'd appeared as a spirit or whether she had looked like an ordinary woman at first.

Frankie stared at the little picture.

Mary's face was flat, neither front-on, nor in profile, and the eyes looked sad – too pale – where the paint had peeled off – not quite meeting her baby's gaze. Frankie leant in realising in that moment that, despite the way she was holding him, it wasn't a baby. Jesus was depicted as a miniature man, with thick coils of auburn hair, wrapped in gold swaddling clothes. No – burial robes. And without knowing why, she crossed herself. 'Please let it be a baby,' she whispered. 'I promise to take care of him – or her,' she added, opening her eyes and glancing furtively around to check no-one had seen her pat her belly.

There was a crunch right behind her – like a smooth-soled shoe – slipping on the gravel.

She spun around.

There was no-one there – just a sudden intake of breath that arrived, from nowhere, to whip a fine grey dust through the pines.

And then it was gone, leaving everything even stiller than before.

She blinked hard and removed her sunglasses but her vision was still not right.

A cool sweat crept over her face.

She crouched down, hung her head between her knees and breathed deeply until she felt better. But when she stood up again, the sky looked wrong – too dark – as if a cloud had passed over the sun – the noise from the cicadas, that she hadn't noticed until that moment – suddenly deafening, while out of the corner of her eye she caught a flicker, as the tail of a lizard disappeared behind a rock.

When they reached the taverna, although Frankie wasn't sure quite what she had been expecting, she was a little disappointed by how dark and dingy it looked. The only sign of any famous circus heritage was a rather shabbily framed flier above the till from 1963 – the ink drawing – of a man leading a bear by a string – scarcely visible behind eleven years of intervening dust.

But the place was perfectly nice. She glanced around; drab whitewashed stone; battered wooden furniture; white paper tablecloths held down with metal clips. And the waiter could not have been more welcoming, she reasoned, sitting up straighter and frowning a little as she glanced over the wipe-clean menu that seemed to serve the same selection as everywhere else they'd eaten that week, breathing in slightly as she contemplated a sixth consecutive day of feta.

The air was hot and too close, their whispered conversation interrupted only by the occasional screech from a little girl in just a nappy and sandals, crouched under a table, trying to catch a cat, while her parents stared straight ahead. On the

other side of the counter, two elderly men played backgammon in the shade of a trellised vine, slumped – in identical fishermen's caps – over rounded tumblers of Metaxa.

Frankie flapped the back of her dress where it had stuck to her neck, and reached for the electric fan before realising it was broken.

The waiter who had shown them to their table was the owner, it turned out, introducing himself as Vasilis in such a soft reedy voice that Frankie had to lean in to hear him properly as he apologised again about the fans, explaining – one hand resting on her elbow – that they were having a bit of trouble with the generator.

He was quite a bit older than them – in his early forties, probably – slight, in a tight-fitting black suit, with an angular face and sparse black hair, slicked-back and combed, carefully, to conceal a prominent waxy forehead, which he wiped with an elaborate display of relief when Callum offered to give him a hand with the generator.

Although Frankie had insisted she would be fine with just a Greek salad, by the time the food arrived she was so hungry that she had to restrain herself from eating all of Callum's moussaka, too, while she waited for him to finish helping Vasilis. She had just started to pick around the edges of it when the kitchen erupted into cheers as all at once the lights came on, the fans burst into life, and the unmistakable growl of Leonard Cohen came booming out of the stereo.

After bringing their change Vasilis lingered a little and struck up conversation once again with Frankie, asking if she had visited the chapel yet and whether she would like his wife, Daphne, to read her palm as a little gift, seeing as it was their honeymoon.

'Oh, no, I...' Frankie flushed, catching Callum's wry smile as he put his sunglasses back on, brushing away a trace of sand from his cheek from where they'd been lying.

'My wife's incredibly superstitious,' he confided, ruffling her hair a little too hard.

But she felt it would be rude to turn the offer down and, no sooner had she agreed, out came Daphne herself. She was not at all as Frankie had imagined – sturdy, forty-odd, about Frankie's height, no make-up, with short permed hair and very flared jeans that almost hid surprisingly small feet, in brown, salt-stained espadrilles.

'Ya, kalimera.' She stared at Frankie, looking her up and down, as she shouted something angrily at her husband in Greek, before turning with curiosity to Callum.

Vasilis smiled, explaining how delighted she was to meet them.

'She says your lines are unusual,' Vasilis observed with a puzzled expression, leaning so close that Frankie could smell the rubbery scent of his aftershave as Daphne sat, perfectly still, staring through her in a trance-like state. 'Very interesting for palm-reading... and so soft! Truly these are not the hands of a farmer's wife.' He laughed.

Daphne glared at him and shifted in her seat, pulling Frankie's index finger so that the joint clicked.

'And this line here...' he explained, as Daphne scratched the side of Frankie's hand '... is for children. You don't have any kids, no?'

Frankie blushed and shook her head, resting one hand on her stomach. She stole a glance at Callum as he sat back to blow a lazy smoke ring, his face to the edge of the sun that was retreating now, behind the awning. But she could tell he was listening.

Before

'It says you will have a child, thanks be to God,' Vasilis added, crossing himself rather half-heartedly as he glanced over at the other table to see whether they'd finished eating.

'Oh, that's good news.' Frankie squeezed Callum's arm. He smiled, almost in spite of himself, and idly examined his own hand while Vasilis and Daphne continued talking in Greek.

'She sees an animal.' Vasilis suppressed a yawn. 'You have some pet? Little dog, maybe?' He checked his watch.

'My husband's a farmer,' said Frankie. 'Like I was saying earlier – about the—'

'Yes, yes.' Vasilis waved away her explanation.

Callum rolled his eyes. 'We should probably be heading back in a bit,' he whispered.

Daphne was watching them carefully through eyes that made no movement. 'No.' She let go of Frankie's hand and slammed the table with her fist, taking a deep breath.

Frankie looked to Vasilis, who seemed agitated. He muttered something to his wife, the words rattling out like bullets. But Daphne refused to interact with him. 'No,' she said again, more calmly now, switching to English and speaking directly to Frankie.

She drew a square with her finger in the air between them. 'Children. One is special – very special for you, Mamá.'

Frankie shrank back in her seat. Her face felt suddenly much too hot.

Vasilis looked confused. 'Special – how do you say – union?' he suggested to Daphne.

'No.'

They waited for her to go on.

'Here.' She jabbed Frankie's hand with her finger. 'This one is for a child – maybe two, although this second one is very soft which means, I don't know, maybe a girl; it's okay, no problem.

But *this* third line…' She pointed it out to Callum and shook her head. 'This very strong special line is broken.'

'What?' Frankie looked down at the side of her palm, staring at the creases beneath her little finger, observing the way the skin still glistened, in the cracks, from the suntan oil, and unsure which lines the woman was referring to. 'What does that mean?'

'It means this child has problem. You have problem.'

'*Ela!*' Vasilis raised his hands and barked something at his wife.

Callum was frowning. He leant in. 'Shall we call it a day? I don't think we should get too involved here.'

Frankie nodded, her face trembling. 'Thank you. I think we'll…' She tried to withdraw her hand but Daphne's grip tightened.

Frankie wrenched her hand away, knocking the table as she stood up, causing the glasses to wobble precariously. She hurried to catch up with Callum, urging him — even though she knew it was pointless — to leave a bigger tip. But as they headed down the hill, she glanced back and raised a hand, just in time to catch the look on Daphne's face before the other woman turned away, leaving Frankie uncertain, for a moment, whether she hadn't caught a glimmer of a smile.

They walked back to the car in silence, Callum a few steps ahead of her. And when they passed the shrine, although Frankie knew it was silly, she shivered.

Callum watched her approach through the wing mirror and started the ignition before she'd got in, revving the engine as she sat down, the scorched leather seat burning the backs of her legs, as she reached automatically behind her, forgetting, again, that there were no seatbelts.

He didn't say anything as they set off.

Before

'That was all a bit weird, wasn't it?' she said.

He didn't reply.

She rested one hand on his leg. 'Are you okay?'

'You've no business bleating all that nonsense about the farm. You don't know what you're talking about.' He wrenched the gear stick too hard so that the tyres skidded.

'What?' She laughed in surprise but her face stung. 'I was just being friendly.'

'It's not friendly, it's fake,' he muttered.

He drove too fast down the hill so that she had to push, hard, with both hands against the broken glove compartment, aware all the time of the pressure against her stomach.

She apologised twice, but he didn't say anything.

'There's no truth in it,' he said eventually, pulling up at the car hire office in the main harbour and walking off before she had a chance to respond. 'It's just rubbish.'

She tried to get him to chat while they waited in the car park for the man to finish his cigarette. 'Can't we just forget it?' She squeezed his hand. 'There's no point arguing on our last day.'

He came round in the end, though, explaining, as they watched the man wade out to inspect the car across a sea of bendy tarmac, that he had just been too hot and had realised that they'd forgotten to tell Ray to pick up that pump they'd ordered. He wouldn't have been able to make a start on it.

'Let's worry about it when we get back,' she said through gritted teeth, the acrid smell leaping from nowhere to surprise her, as she pictured herself, back in the rain, heaving that rusted iron gate through the dense overspill of slurry. 'We're on holiday. Let's—'

'Yeah... last holiday we'll be taking any time soon,' he murmured, getting up to talk to the man, while Frankie stayed seated, trying not to think about the farmhouse – the kitchen – too cold, in their absence, and all closed up, as if it were hiding something.

For they both knew that although there was no further damage to the car, something else had been spoiled by the day. And when they got back to their room, Frankie realised that Callum hadn't once looked at her since the moment they left the taverna.

SCENES FROM CHILDHOOD

April 1998

While the nurse changed her cannula Frankie clenched her fist and looked out the window. The greying maternity block opposite was barely visible against the concrete morning sky, as if it had been cut out of cardboard and stuck on. And as she stared, trying to decipher a face in a tiny rectangle of yellow light, she remembered looking out of one of those windows the day Michael was born – wondering, dimly, whether she would die there too.

She yawned. The pain in her leg and her back was subsiding at least, but the morphine – although it made her drowsy – left her too nauseous to sleep properly. Instead, she felt as if she were already dreaming, lurching between memories that overlapped with the present before sliding back again so that she no longer knew what was now, or then, or still to come.

There was only one constant – in the foreground of her thoughts at all times.

And that was Michael.

Although she had done everything in her power to conceal the fact, Frankie had known, from around the time when Michael first started to talk, that her son was different. Not special, exactly – just different.

It was that Michael seemed to see things that other children didn't see – that other adults didn't see either, for that matter. Not at all like his older brother, John, who had shot into their world with such force that it was as if someone had fired an actual pistol – eight months, to the day, after Frankie and Callum got home from their honeymoon. And she had spent the best part of the following four years – before Michael came along – trying to catch him, as he stampeded and kicked away from her like a startled racehorse.

No, she could never quite find the right words to articulate what it was about Michael. He just seemed, well, sort of spiritual.

He had been rather a strange baby – always listening – watching – suspicious of her. As if he could tell that she was only pretending to know what she was doing. He was small, for a start, and had taken her by surprise when she woke one morning at six, just before the start of lambing season, alarmed to find her body descending rapidly into what would turn out to be a swift, violent labour, three weeks earlier than anticipated.

Frankie felt the light begin to fade.

She closed her eyes.

And after a while a door clicked as she began to lose all sense of her surroundings, save for the bleeping of the machines and the familiar squeak of the nurse's plimsolls as she disappeared down the years to that morning in February when Michael was born.

February 1979

Callum would be gone all day. Frankie knew he wanted to set up the pens early, with the cold weather set to last. She'd barely seen him all week – clearing away the snow – getting the sheds ready for the lambs – repairing the roof.

She leant out the window. The sky was a strange pinkish-grey; the sun – the colour of sour milk. She called down but the yard was bare and through the mist the outbuildings seemed no more substantial than shadows – as if a child had shaded over the scene in chalk.

Surely there must be someone down there? Callum would probably be over in the main barn, she calculated as she tried to focus, her scalp starting to itch with sweat.

But what if he was all the way up on Conway's field already?

She cursed him under her breath as she frantically leafed through the Yellow Pages, wishing she could remember the number for the taxi firm in the village two along from Misselden. The phone rang and rang but no-one answered. She swore loudly and slammed the receiver down, shoving Callum's red Guernsey jumper over her nightie and some old tracksuit bottoms that still fitted.

The pains were starting again – stronger this time. She checked her watch. They were coming quicker. How was she going to get John to Rosemary's?

Hearing music over the crunch of gravel, she was relieved to see the van pull up next to the stable. 'Callum,' she hollered.

'No, it's me.' A red-haired boy climbed out; he looked familiar – in a battered wax jacket that didn't do up properly over his boiler suit – but she couldn't quite place him. 'Everything alright?'

'Have you seen Callum?'

'No, I think he said he's—'

'What about Ray then? Or Jody? I need someone to give me a lift. Now. To the hospital. The baby's coming.'

'Oh, no.' He stepped back, alarmed, wiping his hair out of his eyes as he looked towards the stables for someone to ask. 'I don't know. I could run you over there, I suppose? If that would help, I mean?'

She hesitated, weighing up the situation in her head. 'Could you?' She sighed in relief. 'Thanks. I wouldn't normally…' The pain was coming again. 'I'll be right down,' she shouted, barking out only the essential words, making sure he'd heard her. 'I've got to drop my son at the cottage – the Willows. Come now.'

She stuffed her hospital bag in the pram, grabbing the little white woollen hat that her older sister Bobbi had sent for the baby – still in its wrapping paper. And she hauled John – bewildered and half-asleep – out into the yard. The ground was damp with sleet and snow, and as he ran in tiny steps to keep up with her, she imagined icy water seeping through the thin soles of his Rupert Bear slippers.

As she battled with the gate, she realised she had forgotten to lock up. Her jaw ached and her face felt too hot. She had a sudden image of Callum. Her heart started beating faster.

She stared back at the house, imagining herself – all alone – the baby coming too quickly – being carried into hospital by a stranger – and she looked away so that John wouldn't see her cry. She couldn't do this. What was she thinking?

And then a movement caught her eye.

She looked up – a shape – in the bedroom window.

She stared at the glass. It was too bleary. She wiped her eyes and the shape seemed to step closer. It looked like a woman, watching them.

'Who's that?' Frankie gripped John's hand tighter.

The little boy looked up at her through worried eyes – a line across his cheek from the crease of his pillow.

Pink light flashed on the glass. Frankie jumped. It was just a reflection; she knew that, but her neck prickled with sweat.

She stared hard at the window and blinked away the tears. But the glass darkened before her eyes as a cloud passed over the sun, rubbing out all the pink from the sky and turning everything blank again.

She gasped, clutching her stomach. The pain was shifting gear, ferocious now. She crouched down when it got the better of her, and the moment it started to ease, she flung the gate open and dragged John down the lane, trailing the pram behind them over the ice-hardened mud.

As they waited for Rosemary to come to the door, Frankie tried to take her mind off the mounting pain in her abdomen, staring up at the frosted mush of leaves that had collected in the gap beneath the roof, where the guttering had come away from the stone. 'Oh, hurry *up*, Rosemary.' She scrunched the scrap of paper with the number for the labour ward. And where was that boy? Had he understood? She'd just have to tell Rosemary to get the number to Callum as soon as possible.

A pair of inquisitive eyes peered around the door. 'Good gracious. Mummy forgotten your coat?' The old woman shivered and pulled her purple acrylic dressing gown tight. 'You must be perishing, love.' She turned to Frankie. 'Anyway, I've been dying to tell you—'

'I'm sorry, Rosemary,' Frankie jumped in – keen to get the message out before the pain started again, prising John's fingers from hers in order to physically hand him over to the old woman who had carried on talking as if there had been no interruption.

'Sheila popped by yesterday. You'll never guess. Said that girl from the post office is expecting again. You know the one?'

Frankie shook her head, feeling a powerful muscular shift inside her. Everything in her peripheral vision was darkening. She crouched down.

'You *do*, love: plump; ginger; curls; husband had a to-do with that lady solicitor three down from Maggie Betterick's daughter?'

John was pulling so hard on her arm now that when the van pulled up, music blaring, Frankie thought she might topple over. She wrenched her arm away, dropping the piece of paper as she did so, picturing the worry etched on Callum's face as he headed into driving sleet.

'Sorry about the smell.' The boy leapt out to open the door for her, proceeding to skilfully dismantle the pram without her having to demonstrate. 'I've been fixing the exhaust. We'll just have to have the windows open, if that's okay?'

He held out a hand. 'Don't cry.' He smiled nervously. 'It's going to be fine.'

But she didn't reply.

The van stank of petrol fumes and the back seat was muddy, covered in hair from Lulu, Callum's sheepdog. Frankie grimaced as she hauled herself in.

Piano chords were crashing over a flute or something that was screeching higher and higher. It was Poulenc – one of Callum's tapes – she liked it normally but it was the last thing she needed right now. She put her hands over her ears. 'Turn that off.'

He immediately switched it off, glancing at her anxiously as he checked the back windscreen before reversing the van, fast, down the lane back towards the main road.

Letting the tears fall free, she leant out the window and waved goodbye to John, his furious howl growing smaller and smaller. Not able to bear meeting his gaze, she stared instead up at the gutter – her hot breath leaving a trail, like smoke, through the cold silence – as she concentrated on not letting her body give birth in the van and imagining herself stuffing the leaves into the end of the pipe where they belonged.

When Michael was born, an hour and a half later, the midwife sounded almost disappointed to observe that he was a lovely healthy boy as Frankie lay there, finally numb, like an old wrinkled balloon the day after the celebration.

She watched him coming towards her in the midwife's outstretched hands – his little grey body defenceless to the onslaught of the morning. His hair was dark, his face squashed and alien – eyes glued shut. And as she fed him – her body seemingly remembering, without understanding, what to do – she noticed a bright red birthmark, like a crushed loganberry, just above his left hip.

Afterwards, as the midwife stood by the weighing scales, enfolding him in a worn white towel, the heap of bloody placenta dumped unceremoniously on the counter, she reminded Frankie of a butcher, wrapping a joint of lamb just before it is placed, fat and squeaking, on a thin polystyrene dish.

Frankie left the ward that afternoon, before having been officially discharged, knowing she couldn't leave John any longer.

A couple of nurses were hovering around the television in the corridor and as she hauled herself stiffly out of bed and over to the window, she overheard the reporter explain that the gravediggers in Liverpool had agreed to call off their strike. She stared down at the car park, picturing a body, dumped, in the snow.

Kneeling carefully to gather her belongings, she caught the start of Callaghan's sentence but the jeering was so loud by the time he'd finished speaking that it was impossible to know what he'd been trying to say.

No-one seemed to notice her shuffling away.

She sat, awkward and shivering, on a wall near the bus stop. The bin was overflowing and a crust of icy footprints had started to melt, exposing a dirty trail along the pavement of crisp packets and Mars bar wrappers and cigarette ends. Whenever she put any of her weight down, she felt a thick, heavy ache in her perineum that seemed to shoot right through her, up to her jaw. And when she stood up too quickly, seeing silent headlights in the fog, it was as if her thighs had come unstuck from her torso. She leant against the pram as she edged towards the bus, like a survivor of an explosion emerging from the rubble.

May 1998

Frankie had been in hospital for three weeks after the fire before the feeling returned fully in her left leg. The physiotherapist said it was a miracle she'd survived, nicknaming her Lazarus with a dissatisfied sneer as she stood, hands on hips, scrutinising every movement of the trainee nurse who was silently disinfecting Frankie's wounds.

'Not had one as bad as this since that fourteen-year-old lad, have we? Climbed up a crane for some drunken bet; ended up falling twenty-two feet on to the roof of a JCB. Broke every single vertebra in his back.' She gave a little snort. 'And guess who had to break the news to Mum that he'd never walk again?'

Although Frankie did guess, it didn't make her feel any better. If anything, she detected an unwelcome note of opprobrium in the physiotherapist's whole approach, as if she were suggesting that Frankie had jumped for the sheer hell of it – just to make everyone's life a little more complicated. And although Frankie was aware that she, herself, was probably coming across as surly and unco-operative, especially when she howled out as the nurse accidentally knocked her ankle – in reality, it was because she was terrified, despite the physiotherapist's reassurance to the contrary, that her leg would be permanently damaged.

She was filled, all day and all night, with an unabating rage at her son, made all the more unbearable by the fact that she was finding it so difficult to move her leg. It was like a poison that had gathered in wells inside her, and she couldn't shake it around or shift its weight to dilute it. She feared it would finish her off.

But of course, she couldn't say anything to anyone else about any of that.

And so, instead, she closed her eyes and pretended she was somewhere else, finding herself dragged, almost against her will, back to that time when the boys were little.

He must have been about two – Michael – when he first saw it – two and a half, maybe. Yes, she calculated. They would have been in Oxford a year or so by then.

It all felt such a blur – that period after she left Callum and the farm. They'd stayed with Bobbi initially, near Cardigan, and then spent a few weeks along the coast in New Quay, in a run-down seaside B&B with carpet on the walls in the foyer. Callum had still found them, of course, as he always would, although it didn't take him as long in those days. So they'd gone back to the farm after that. And hadn't left again until Michael turned one.

But it was those weeks in Wales that had shown her that life could be different. And it was there that she had made the decision to move back to Oxford to be nearer her father, as soon as she was strong enough. She and Bobbi had never been especially close to him; both privately blamed him for their mother's decision to leave them, a few days before Frankie's thirteenth birthday. But it was reassuring to know he'd be there, if she needed him, in an emergency.

And once she'd spotted a place in East Oxford – an unremarkable red-brick end-of-terrace with a garden that looked out towards the car plant – he'd surprised her by agreeing not only to help her get the mortgage but also to pay the first few months until she found her feet.

It had felt so safe – so warm and light and empty, at first, after the loaded darkness of the farm – not to mention the constant worry of seeing her husband around every corner. And yet how she would grow to hate that house, too, and what took place there, with more and more intensity, as the years of John and Michael's childhood gradually slipped away.

October 1981

Frankie was sitting on the spare bed with Michael on her knee – the door open – to keep one ear on John, still deep-sea diving in the bath. She had agreed to read one last story before she put Michael down in his cot that he was already beginning to outgrow, she observed again guiltily, but she had only just started working again – as a receptionist in the GP surgery round the corner from John's school – and hadn't yet the means to replace it.

When she closed the book, Michael turned to face her, reaching up to put his arms around her neck. He was warm from the bath and his skin smelt of camomile and talcum powder.

'Right.' She pulled away. 'Time for bed.' She kissed him on the forehead and he laughed, placing his hands on either side of her face. He pulled her close, his eyes bright. And then he kissed her on the nose and burst out laughing again, throwing his head back and slapping her on the cheeks.

She laughed, pretending to be cross. 'What a rascal.'

He did it again and gazed, unblinking, into her eyes.

She looked away, momentarily afraid to look too long into those eyes.

It felt dangerous to love anyone with that intensity.

When one day they would be sure to leave you.

She buried her face in his chest so he didn't see her tears.

'Who's that?' he whispered.

She looked up.

He had stopped laughing. His eyes were still glowing but he was pointing at something just behind her. And to see the little face lit up like that from a different angle made it look, in that moment, as if it belonged to someone else.

She turned around to see what he was looking at.

The landing was in darkness.

She looked down at him, her pulse raised.

He was staring tenderly at the absence.

Frankie flushed. She stood up. 'It's bedtime now, Michael,' she said loudly, her eyes flickering back to the staircase as she lifted him into the cot.

He sat very still, his little spidery hands gripping the wooden slats of the cot. He was smiling – a strange, beatific smile, his dark eyes resting on the space above her shoulder.

And then he nodded.

'I'm talking to my mummy,' he said.

Frankie felt a twinge in her chest and she lay him down, too firmly.

'John,' she called, trying to ignore the waver in her voice. 'It's time to get out now.' She could hear him splashing and blowing bubbles with his snorkel. She went into the bathroom and snatched the plug out, accidentally catching his foot with the thin chain so that he cried out in annoyance.

And then she went back into the bedroom, closing the door behind her to block out John's screams of protest.

She kissed Michael on the top of his head. 'Goodnight, little one. Let's lie down now.'

"Night, Mummy.' He pulled the blanket to his chin.

Frankie glanced back at him as she closed the door and noticed a little flutter of his hand as he blew her a kiss.

It happened again, though, not long after that.

And by the time Michael had reached his third birthday these visions were happening frequently enough to occupy much of Frankie's thoughts during the daytime, uncertain, as ever, of what was to come after the sun had gone down.

She had come to dread the evenings. It didn't happen when John was there but he never wanted to have stories with Michael. She couldn't blame him. He was almost seven by then and it was pretty much the only time in the day that he had on his own with her. Besides, of course he had no interest in that little Noah's Ark picture book. He wanted her to read things that he couldn't manage alone. They were halfway through *The Ghost of Thomas Kempe*; she remembered – for although she wasn't to know it at the time – it would turn out to be the last book they would read together in that way. But Frankie was also a little afraid to admit that she wanted John in Michael's room for her benefit – not his.

One time it happened it had shaken her insides and she found afterwards that, no matter what she ate, she couldn't keep anything down. It felt like a form of reflux. On the days after an incident, while John was at school and Michael at playgroup, her mouth tasted of thick bile.

On that particular evening Michael had lain down, quiet and calm, in his cot as usual. She had leant over him and kissed him goodnight, but before going to John, she listened a few moments at Michael's door.

And after a while she heard Michael whispering.

She pushed the door open a crack.

Michael was standing straight – his back to her – at the end of his cot, staring up at the bookcase.

'Don't cry,' he said solemnly. 'Mummy's here.'

'Who are you talking to, Michael?' Frankie's voice came out too loud as she tried to swallow the saliva-coated panic that she felt rising from the back of her throat.

He didn't turn around. It was as if his eyes were fixed on something.

'I'm talking to the lady.'

Frankie tried to block the back of her throat with her tongue. 'Lie down,' she growled, managing to wait until she was downstairs before giving in to her body in the way it so violently needed her to.

After she had bleached the sink, she threw the remains of the casserole in the bin and drank a bottle of red wine instead – glass by glass by glass.

Her throat burnt.

She thought she heard footsteps outside Michael's bedroom that evening, as she did on so many occasions that would follow. But each time she went into the hallway to check, there was never anything there. And yet, that particular night, when she lugged her weary frame up the stairs to bed, having very nearly fallen asleep in front of *Dynasty*, she hesitated for a second, before deciding to leave the landing light on.

June 1998

In the end, the insurance company did pay out. But not the full amount. And thirty per cent less than she had been led to believe she would be able to claim (when she had paid for the damned thing in the first place) in the highly unlikely event of precisely such an eventuality coming to pass.

There was practically nothing left of the house – nothing to rebuild even if she had wanted to. Not that she did, Frankie reflected, wiping her eyes as John helped her out of the car and over to the hospital garden for her first outpatients' session with the physiotherapist.

In fact, the very thought of waiting any time at all – let alone the eighteen months that she had been quoted – to build something that she didn't really want anyway, in exactly the spot in which her son had left her for dead, filled her with a deep sense of revulsion.

She leant heavily on the crutches, while across the car park a boy with a wobbly pink helium balloon followed his father into the maternity unit.

Scarlet peonies lined the path to the small, enclosed courtyard garden, and as they approached she noticed a dead pigeon in the flower bed, positioned so that its body lay on the earth, and its head – with the neck perfectly twisted – on the path, its cheek resting on the stone, as though someone had placed it there as an offering.

April 1983

A year or so after those first disturbances, Michael started waking in the night, screaming – a piercing wail that Frankie mistook at first for foxes mating by the bins below her bedroom window. The first time it happened she sat up suddenly, still half-asleep, disoriented. It must be him, she thought, hesitating as she slid her feet into her slippers because he had rarely cried until then, apart from as a baby, of course. And since she'd moved him out of the cot, he usually just pattered across the landing if he woke in the night, climbing into her bed without a word, before going back to sleep.

This was different.

Children shouldn't cry like that.

How on earth could John sleep through that noise?

She pushed softly against Michael's door and the moment it clicked open the noise stopped. She looked into the darkened room. She could only make out a black, formless shape in his bed. She leant over his little sleeping body, feeling for his arms – stretched aside like wings. His breathing was calm. She didn't know why but something made her rest one hand, very gently, against his cheek, to check it was warm.

'A bad dream,' it turned out, as he calmly chatted to his brother in that serious little voice the next morning at the kitchen table, while earnestly chewing his muesli.

'Fire, fire.'

It was always exactly the same from then on. He would think that the fire would get them all. He would be frightened.

It was his fault again. And Mummy was hurt. But Michael would be sorry.

Frankie always felt the same rush of relief that she hadn't imagined the whole thing but she never said anything, in all that time. She would just stand at the window, soothing her hands in the hot soapy water of the washing-up bowl – anything to avoid those pebbly grey eyes that never seemed to reflect the light truthfully – like a memorial left there to prevent her from forgetting the man to whom – in the eyes of the Father – she was still married.

Some nights she woke up and rushed into him, convinced she could smell smoke herself. Other nights she managed to ignore it entirely, as if she had consciously decided to sleep over the noise or her mind had given permission to her tired old body to rest just a little longer before heaving itself upright again to face the new day.

It was Frankie's sister, Bobbi, who was the first other one to witness it first-hand, as it were.

Frankie had tried to hide her astonishment, as she turned into the road one Tuesday lunchtime – having picked Michael up from playgroup as usual on her way back from the surgery – to see Bobbi's battered red Fiesta parked outside the house. She couldn't have driven all the way over from Wales?

Her sister stuck her head out the window and pressed on the horn as Frankie approached. 'Well, fancy seeing you here,' she drawled. She was artfully dishevelled in Frankie's old denim jacket, and impossibly long-legged when she climbed out; Frankie noticed that her sister's heavy kohl eyeliner – always so carefully applied – was smudged, today, at the edges. Bobbi's gaze landed with secret delight on her younger sister's slightly expanded waist; her smile was taut – chatter too breezy.

'Where are the girls?' Frankie had asked.

'Al's mum's there. Although I don't see why he can't deal with them on his own, for once,' Bobbi had snapped.

'Well, it's the middle of the school week. Isn't he—'

'Oh, don't *you* start.' Bobbi reached down to help unpack the bags of groceries stuffed underneath the pushchair as Frankie carried the still-sleeping child upstairs.

But although Frankie felt a little apprehensive, she secretly welcomed the chance to have some company for the evening, knowing that her sister would soften as the afternoon wore on.

And Bobbi was sorry to turn up out of the blue like that. She'd be out of Frankie's hair first thing in the morning, she had promised. Besides, she had to be getting back for the girls.

It had been a stupid row about that woman again – 'Yes, the English teacher.' All blown out of proportion. She knew he was telling the truth this time but she just couldn't help bringing it up whenever they argued. 'I'd be able to handle it, I think, if she wasn't so... so fucking smiley,' Bobbi had scowled, kneeling down to root around in the cupboard for a balsamic vinegar substitute. 'About as much edge as a Victoria sponge. Less, possibly,' she murmured, checking the label on a jar of dried basil. 'Dresses like a mum in an OshKosh catalogue.'

She stood up and leant against the counter, deep in thought. 'So everyone else thinks she's really nice, obviously.' She swept her hair out of her eyes. 'And there I am – can't say anything – the only one who can see she's an absolute first-prize manipulative bitch.' She wrinkled her nose. 'It's disappointing, more than anything, to think he'd have such poor taste.'

It wasn't until later that Frankie realised her sister hadn't had anywhere else to go. And she was ashamed when Bobbi reminded her that they hadn't seen each other since that time Frankie came to stay with her when Michael was a baby.

Frankie left Michael with Bobbi that afternoon while she went to collect John from school. When she got back, she changed out of her work things and put on some make-up, trying out a corally lipstick that she'd bought months back but still hadn't opened. She looked a little better. She frowned back at herself, peering closer at the shadows under her eyes. But Callum was right; whatever shade she tried, lipstick always aged her. She wiped her mouth with the back of her hand and went into Michael's room to make up the spare bed.

She sat down on the bed and closed her eyes, tempted to lie down for an hour or so.

And just as she felt her head start to fall forwards, there was a hand on her shoulder.

She jumped.

Michael was standing right next to her.

'Oh, you gave me a fright.' She laughed and got up quickly, reaching for the clean pillowcases. 'It's very kind of you to let Auntie Bobbi go in your room tonight.'

He went over to the window seat and started to pull things out of his toy box.

As she struggled with the duvet cover, she watched him carefully select Dodo – a threadbare orange elephant that he'd had since he was a baby. It had been a gift from Rosemary, their neighbour, on the farm.

He lay it on the pillow of the spare bed. 'Auntie Bobbi can cuddle Dodo,' he explained.

There was something about the way the light was shining behind him that made his eyes look black – opaque – Callum's eyes, as her sister would later corroborate, not for the first time, to Frankie's growing sense of dismay. She swallowed and leant down to kiss him on the top of his head before dragging his cot into John's room. 'I love you,' she said, after a momentary pause.

But when Frankie attempted, that evening, to pick up their conversation where they'd left off, Bobbi had promptly changed the subject, preoccupying herself instead with an elaborate caramelised onion tart recipe she'd cut out of the *Observer* magazine several weeks earlier.

The conversation still stuttered and their laughter felt forced – even after Bobbi opened a second bottle of wine. So Frankie suggested, after they'd finally finished eating, that they move into the living room where it was a bit comfier.

'Sorry I've not got much chat.' Frankie gave a deep yawn. 'Michael's been waking in the night quite a bit.'

Bobbi raised one eyebrow but said nothing.

'Bad dreams, I think,' Frankie ventured. 'But it's exhausting, isn't it?'

'If it's any consolation, it does get easier.' She stretched out her legs. 'Sort of,' she added, examining her long narrow feet with dissatisfaction. 'They're so young still, aren't they? It must be hard being away from their dad.'

Frankie frowned, fiddling with one of the cushions; a button had come loose.

'It's different for boys. Everyone says so. They need male role models.'

'Hmm... I'm not sure all role models are that helpful,' Frankie muttered.

Bobbi pulled a face. 'I'm obviously not letting anyone off the hook. But nothing's perfect. And it's not exactly easy on your own either, is it?'

'I don't know.' Frankie pulled the thread tighter, accidentally snapping it so that the button sprang off.

Bobbi stared at her, a challenge in her eyes that reminded Frankie of their dad. 'Come on, Frankie.' She reached for her glass. 'We *all* told you it would be hard work. You wouldn't listen—'

'I didn't have a choice,' Frankie said, a darkness building inside.

There were just too many years that had passed between them for there to be any shared chronology anymore – any family, she realised, draining her wine glass.

She could tell that Bobbi sensed it too, especially when she begged Frankie to stay up for five more minutes, when she saw her sister's expression. 'You still haven't told me where you're up to with the café idea? I'm still keen, you know, in principle. Last time we spoke, you'd spotted a place in Llangranog or somewhere, hadn't you?'

'Oh, no, that was just a silly pipe dream.' Frankie looked away – a fleeting vision of herself on an icy beach, backed against a wall, an implacable tide snatching at her wet hair.

Bobbi fell back on safer ground after that, beginning again to narrate the handful of childhood stories that featured their mother before she had left – tales that they hadn't told for a long time but which they had nevertheless both silently determined to commit to memory – like the words of a prayer – for the comfort that they brought in their sharing.

And although she joined in, Frankie had to look away at one point, feeling self-conscious. They had been doing it for so many years now that she felt guilty to admit that she no longer remembered which of the details were real. And which were the embellishments of a much beloved and necessary ritual.

When Frankie heard a noise that night, in the back of her head, she almost managed to convince her body to ignore it. But then she heard movement and got up quickly, grabbing her dressing gown from the hook on the door, shy all of a sudden when she remembered they had a visitor.

And then there she was – Bobbi – cowering at the top of the stairs – her long dark hair, wild, and sticking up all over the place, like when they were teenagers and used to backcomb it. Her face was sweaty. She looked straight through Frankie.

'Bobbi?' Frankie edged towards her sister. 'Are you alright?'

Bobbi stared at her in terror. And then, when the words had registered, something in her face seemed to drop. 'Where am I?' She looked all around her and shook her hands as if to physically release herself from the grip of the night. She seemed to regain a sense of normality and gave a funny laugh. 'Sorry, I don't know what…'

She folded her arms in embarrassment and patted her hair, now conscious of her surroundings. 'I had a terrible dream.'

She laughed again. But she reached out with one hand to steady herself against the wall. 'I had to get the girls. We couldn't get out.'

Frankie felt her face grow hot.

Bobbi looked down at her hands as if to check she was still there. 'Ridiculous, isn't it?' She turned as if to go back into the room. But then she stopped and stared straight at Frankie, with urgency. 'I couldn't get to them.'

Frankie's hands stiffened and she caught a trace of a scent – like petrol. She tried to breathe more slowly, through her mouth.

Bobbi was just about to speak but then she stopped, her eyes focused on something just behind Frankie.

Frankie spun around. She felt light-headed and her heart was suddenly beating too fast. 'Oh, Michael,' she said, relieved, grabbing the banister as she crouched down to hug him to her.

'I'm sorry,' whispered Bobbi. 'Did we wake you up?'

Michael was watching Bobbi closely, his head resting on Frankie's shoulder. He was clutching Dodo, his little orange elephant.

Bobbi reached down and ruffled his hair. 'Let's all go back to sleep, shall we?' Her voice shook a little, as if she weren't quite convinced of the wisdom of her own suggestion.

But Michael ignored her. He wriggled free of Frankie's embrace and stared straight at his mother before looking down at the little toy elephant in his hands.

'The fire was on Dodo,' he said.

Frankie stared at him, wondering whether she was still asleep. 'What did you say?'

'I needed to save Dodo.'

And then, when he finally dared to look back up at her, she saw something in his eyes that she couldn't unsee. It was a look of challenge. As if he wanted to show her that he knew she'd betrayed him and that he'd discovered the truth for himself.

And she couldn't think of anything to say to him.

But she nodded.

Bobbi left straight after breakfast – their conversation less stilted than before, and safe, at least, without any reference to the night.

And although, for a few months, they called each other more often than before, things eventually got back to normal. Bobbi and Al seemed to get their lives back on track and Frankie's evenings became gradually shorter as the boys grew up, but they were just so far apart that it was hard to ever really make plans to meet up. Until it got to the point where both sisters simply stopped calling, knowing – all the same – that if they needed anything they would just pick up the phone, tacitly accepting the settlement as the years passed them by – a sort of benevolent truce.

Yes, even if life had turned out quite differently – setting aside the horrors of John and Olivia's wedding, Frankie would one day reflect, a grim taste in her mouth – she wondered whether she would have seen that much more of her sister anyway, after all that.

June 1998

At the far end of the courtyard, a gardener was deadheading a rose. And as Frankie and John sat down on the rounded iron bench to wait for the physiotherapist, she noticed that the rockery discreetly hid a water feature, giving the impression that the roses were weeping too.

'Have you heard from Michael?' she said to John.

John shook his head and looked away. 'I hope he's okay, Mum.'

She resisted the urge to tell him to stop fiddling with the car keys.

'Liv's still adamant she doesn't want him at the wedding,' he said.

'Perhaps you could ask him to play something?'

Frankie gave a little snarl as she spotted the physiotherapist in the distance and hurriedly wiped her eyes.

The physiotherapist didn't acknowledge them as she approached. Still scribbling on her clipboard, she apologised for keeping them waiting and shot Frankie an antiseptic smile before commanding her to get up and show them all what this leg of hers was really made of.

Frankie was through with them – all of them, she decided, trying to force her disobedient left foot to swing in something resembling the circular pattern that the physiotherapist had demonstrated so effortlessly. And they could try as hard as they liked to fob her off but they weren't getting rid of her that easily. She was alive. And she'd make her damned leg work again if it was the last thing she did.

She'd been doing a lot of thinking lately. And had come to the realisation that she needed to do things *her* way from now on. She had lost everything. Well, she reflected, watching the ankle shudder in a weak imitation of the loop she'd intended – everything in the house, of course, but she hadn't quite lost everything. She still had herself. They couldn't take that away from her.

And from now on she was going to use whatever little of anything she had left before they took the rest of it – her money, undoubtedly, but far more precious even than that: her time. Starting – she decided grimly, as she set about retraining the big toe – by getting back in touch with Omar.

She thought back to that lovely evening in the meadow and tried to picture them together now, with her leg like this. She frowned, feeling the tears building again. Maybe it would be better to wait until her leg had recovered.

She was going to try a bit harder with Bobbi, too. She had been meaning to remind John and Olivia to invite Bobbi and Al to the wedding. But perhaps she should also go and stay a couple of days. These things were important, she realised now. She should make the effort before it was too late.

But she had plenty of time. What was that irritating thing the physiotherapist kept repeating, as if there were any other way of doing anything? 'One step at a time, Lazarus.'

And in the meantime, she'd treat herself to a nice holiday. She had a couple of ideas already on where she might like to go.

'Maybe when you're signing the register or something?' she suggested at the end of the session, when John offered to bring the car closer. 'Do you think she'd prefer that?'

February 1985

It was for his sixth birthday that Michael had requested a clarinet.

Frankie had just got back from picking the boys up from Sunday School, having enjoyed a whole hour, uninterrupted, in the garden. It was cold but bright and the daffodils were out already. After hanging up the washing she had decided to dust off a picnic chair from the shed and took her book and a cup of coffee outside. But by the time they got home the sun had vanished and in its place rain clouds were assembling.

So she asked Michael to give her a hand bringing the washing back in.

He sat down, deep in thought, on the picnic chair, feet resting on the laundry basket in front of him. As she passed the clothes down from the line he folded them neatly in the basket, leaving a corner for the pegs.

'Mum,' he said finally. 'Did Jesus play when he was little?'

'What?' She fumbled with the corner of the sheet, dropping a peg. 'What do you mean?'

'Did he go to school? Playgroup or something?'

'Oh, I don't think so. He probably would have stayed at home most of the time. With his mum,' she added, a little doubtfully. 'Or learnt things at church – well, you know – not church, obviously – but at the temple – the synagogue.'

'But I mean, did he play? Like tennis?'

She laughed. 'I doubt it.' They didn't really play tennis in those days.'

'Football, then?'

She clamped the corner of the ice-cold sheet between her teeth as she tried to think of something to say. 'Yes, I expect so. Now, your birthday's coming up. I was wondering if you'd had any ideas of what you'd like?'

'I already told you: a Bananaman lunchbox.'

'Yes, I mean apart from that.'

'A clarinet, then.'

She stared at him.

'Please.'

'A clarinet?'

He nodded patiently. 'I had a go on one at Sunday School. The lady who does the music showed me. It's in the woodwind family,' he explained, as if she were the child.

'Oh...' she said, a little flustered, and ashamed to admit that she wasn't sure what it looked like – let alone sounded like. She suddenly heard Callum's voice in her head and wondered why that particular line came to mind right then: 'not exactly a crap mum,' he used to say, 'just inexperienced.'

'Well, I'll have to think about that.'

'Mum?'

She hesitated. 'Yes, Michael?'

'Did Jesus's mum have a job?'

'Well,' she bristled. 'Sort of. She was in charge of looking after *him*. That's quite an important job, isn't it, Michael? Come on, it's about to chuck it down in a minute. Let's go in.'

He stood up but still looked puzzled.

'What is it, Michael?' she snapped.

He raised one hand and brought it down emphatically. 'So, did Jesus have packed lunch then? Or school lunch?'

She popped into the music shop on the High Street a couple of weeks later, in her lunch hour, but after learning the prices she thought no more of it.

On Michael's birthday he came into her room early, dragging a half-sleeping John behind him so that when Frankie opened her eyes fully, she was surprised to find the two of them sitting patiently on the end of her bed.

'Is it time for my present, Mum?'

When Michael opened the Narnia book, the lunchbox, the game of Happy Families and the harmonica he was pleased and hugged Frankie, hard, around the neck. But after breakfast, he turned to her solemnly. 'Do I have to wait until I'm seven for my clarinet?'

'Your what? Oh, the clarinet. I'd forgotten all about it, Michael.'

He looked down at his empty cereal bowl.

'You know they're not toys. They're very expensive.'

He gave a tiny nod.

She hesitated. 'Maybe we could see about borrowing one from school?'

He sniffed but didn't look at her.

'What is it, Michael? You look a bit worried.'

'I don't want to go to school today,' he whispered.

'Hey, come here.' She crouched down and hugged him, waving John upstairs to go and brush his teeth. 'It's your birthday; it'll be fun. You've got to go to school *today*.'

'I don't know who's my friend.' His shoulders heaved and he clung more tightly.

'What do you mean? You've got lots of friends. And you've got me and John and—'

'I don't mean that. I mean at school. I'm not like everyone else. They don't play with me.'

She clasped him to her and looked out of the window as she tried to think of something to say. She stroked his hair. 'Look, Michael,' she ventured. 'It takes time to make friends; why don't we invite someone to come and play at the weekend?'

He shook his head. 'They're not the same.'

'Well, no-one's the same as anyone else.' She patted his back, checking her watch; they'd have to go in a minute. 'We're all different; it's what makes us special.'

'That's not true. John's not different. You're not different.'

She looked at him warily.

'I hear this voice, Mummy.'

She felt a chill run through her. 'What kind of voice?' she said evenly.

'I don't know. It's a man's voice. When I'm asleep.'

She hugged him tighter so he wouldn't be able to see the expression on her face.

'It's scary. Can you make it stop?'

She nodded, trying to think of something to say and after a while she pulled away.

'Right. Let's get going. We'll... we'll talk about this in a minute. On the way to school. But can you run and brush your teeth? And perhaps we could, maybe, save up for a clarinet,' she found herself saying. 'For next year.'

He clasped his hands very tightly around her neck and looked at her, his eyes wide. He wiped away the tears. 'Can we? Really?' His voice was feverish. 'How long is it until my next birthday?'

'It's a year, Michael.'

'Okay. I can start saving up now. I've got a whole year to save up.' His voice grew calm again. 'And if you save up too, together we can have enough money to buy it.'

And then, hearing John coming back, Michael got up from

the table and headed for the stairs. 'I know they cost more than a hundred pounds – even the ones made out of plastic,' he called out behind him. 'I asked the lady at church. But we can't get a plastic one, Mum. I need one that's made of wood. She said the wood ones sound different.'

John bent down to put on his shoes. When they heard Michael going into the bathroom, he said, 'I think some kids were laughing at him at lunch yesterday.'

'Were they? That's awful. Where were the teachers? Who was it?'

'Just some stupid kids in Year Four. Me and Dominic told them to leave him alone. They're always picking on someone. Don't worry. We'll keep an eye on him today in the playground.' He stood up.

'Thank you,' she said, with a deep sense of relief, squeezing him so hard by the arm that he cried out in annoyance.

After that, Michael had talked, quite matter-of-factly and with surprising regularity, about his clarinet. Every so often he would organise a fundraising activity – usually sales of chocolate cornflake cakes or fresh orange juice that he and John squeezed laboriously by hand and poured into tiny paper cups that Frankie brought back from the dispensary.

He would line them up on a creaky, paint-stained trellis table that had been left in the garden shed by the previous owners. And he would stand on the pavement, just outside the front door, with an old biscuit tin covered in Christmas wrapping paper for the money. Occasionally a passer-by would take pity on the earnest little boy, standing there, whatever the weather, with his carefully annotated diagram of a clarinet taped to the tabletop, and would spare a few coins, here and there, after speaking to him about his musical ambitions.

Afterwards, he would sit at the kitchen table, marking the new tally on his sheet – grimly undeterred. 'Just two hundred and seventy-nine pounds to go,' he announced one evening, a few weeks before his seventh birthday, 'because I've got to give at least ten pounds to the poor.'

The Sunday before his birthday, he had been out all afternoon collecting, and by the time Frankie had finished clearing up all the Lego it was later than she realised.

She opened the front door to call him in and was startled to find him standing right there in front of her on the doorstep.

'Come in, it's getting dark.'

His cheeks were purple from the cold, making his eyes too bright and she couldn't quite read his expression. He was clutching something behind his back.

'What have you got—'

He let out a strange laugh – too high-pitched, so that it sounded almost robotic. 'Don't be cross.'

'What is it?'

He unclamped his fingers so slowly that she stepped back, half-expecting a cockroach to run out at her.

She stared.

It was a wad of folded money.

'Where d'you get that?' She snatched it out of his hand.

'Someone gave it to me.'

'Who?' She yanked him inside by the sleeve, slamming the door behind them as she turned the key.

'Where's John? Who gave it to you?'

'It was just a man,' he said, looking away.

'What man?' She grabbed him by the wrists. 'Someone we know?'

'I don't know.' He wriggled away from her and started to

unbutton his grey duffel coat, struggling, as he always did, with the top button.

'What did he look like? Here, let me…' She untangled the toggle from its little leather loop and hurried to the back door, pulling the bolt across.

She ran up the stairs. 'John,' she hollered. 'Come down now. It's nearly dinner.' She went into her bedroom and over to the window.

She looked down.

The street was empty.

She drew the curtains, sat on the bed, and with shaking hands counted eleven five-pound notes that were soft – well-worn – one of them so ragged that someone had seen fit to reinforce it with a sliver of Sellotape – before reaching for the Agatha Christie on her bedside table to hide them – flat – between its pages, like a flower press.

Michael was sitting on the floor of the living room, elbow deep in a box of Lego. 'Mum, will you play—'

She held him tight by the arm.

'Ow – let go.'

'Who was he, this man? What did he look like?'

'I can't remember.' He pulled away, reaching into the box again and started to root around. 'We need another black one with two things on for the drawbridge.'

'Michael.' She snatched the box away from him. 'What did he say?'

'Don't shout.' He bowed his head and started to cry. 'I promised I wouldn't tell you.'

'Tell me what?' She could feel her face tremble. She took a deep breath and tried to speak more gently. 'Did he look like…' She swallowed hard. 'Was it Daddy?'

Michael shook his head, too fast, but he didn't say anything.

'Are you telling the truth?'
'I don't know.'
'Mum!' John was calling her from upstairs.
Gritting her teeth, she shoved the box of Lego back in the cupboard. It wasn't closed properly and all the pieces fell out the other end.
'Mum!' John shouted again.
'What is it?' she screamed back.
Michael cowered.
'What's for dinner?' John shouted.
Michael got up. 'Why do you have to spoil everything?' he whispered.
She heard him crying as he climbed the stairs to his bedroom.
And as she heaved herself to her feet she noticed a little pool of urine – on the carpet in front of her – in the place where Michael had been trying to talk to her.

They chose the clarinet together.
She held back as Michael chatted to the shopkeeper and watched him empty his bag of cash, mainly in twenty-pence pieces, straight on to the glass counter so that Frankie could write a cheque to cover the difference.
He already knew which reeds to get for the mouthpiece, choosing the slightly thicker ones, explaining, in detail, how much he preferred the sound and was determined that he would soon enough be ready for them. He knew how to clean it too, and how to apply that special balm that came included, in a tube, like lip salve, for greasing the cork joints between the limbs of the instrument.
The shopkeeper opened up the black plastic case for Michael to inspect the taut, bright blue velvet inside. And Frankie

noticed the way her son's eyes shone as the man placed the components of the shiny clarinet into the specially moulded grooves, reminding his baffled mother of the importance of opening it the right way up, 'like a toolbox, so you don't damage the keys.'

When they got home, he disappeared straight into his bedroom.

She looked up through the banisters as she pulled on her wellies to go out into the garden and noticed that Michael had left his door open.

Outside, she knelt down and pulled on her thick gardening gloves, reaching over to tug out the stringy weeds that had rooted themselves, with grim permanence, in the cracks between the paving stones that she had so lovingly restored shortly after they had moved in.

And when Michael started to play, softly, and with a sense of control that surprised her – just simple scales and arpeggios at first – the sound carried all the way through the house and out into the garden.

She sat back on her heels and looked up at his window.

And then, after a while, she got up, taking care not to make too much noise and went back into the house through the kitchen. She stood in the hallway, a fist of weeds in her hand, like a withered bouquet.

He stopped, as if he had been waiting for her.

And then he started to play something serious. It was a haunting, woody sound. She wasn't sure whether she recognised it but it was arresting in its melancholy and when he reached the higher notes it reminded her of something from a long time before that she couldn't quite place – very simple – caught somewhere between a lullaby and a prayer.

She looked down at her mud-encrusted gloves and wiped

her eye carefully with the little space of arm above her left wrist.

And then she sat down very quietly on the bottom stair, wishing, almost in spite of herself, that she had someone with whom to share that moment, as she closed her eyes and listened – really listened – to her son.

August 1998

Frankie had been staying at Olivia's flat in Southampton ever since she got out of hospital. John and Olivia had got engaged the previous summer on holiday in Tuscany with Brian and Susanna Whitaker, Olivia's parents. And although Frankie felt awful about imposing, Olivia had insisted, rather kindly in retrospect, that she stay with her and John for a few weeks until she found somewhere suitable.

It was a 'no-brainer', apparently, according to Olivia. 'Mummy always says to Daddy, "What's the point in having a two-bed – smack bang in the nicest part of town – if you don't even use the second room?"'

Although the spare room was small, it was on the ground floor, which made life considerably easier for Frankie. And Olivia kept the whole flat inhumanly neat, surprising Frankie, when she arrived, at just how quickly she felt at home there. There was a sack of dried lavender in the wardrobe that Olivia had brought back from a farm they'd visited in Tuscany, planning to sort it into individual bags for the favours, Frankie had gleaned from the detailed wedding rotas already taped to the kitchen cupboards. So Frankie found that her clothes and her few remaining belongings quickly absorbed a strong scent of lavender, deciding, after a while, that she rather liked it.

During the week, John was out at work and Olivia at college, studying for her LPC, and they spent most weekends at Brian and Susanna's near Winchester, so Frankie saw delightfully little of anyone. And she caught herself one evening, somewhere around the forty-second photograph of an increasingly suntanned Olivia leaning, backlit, into fields of said lavender, thinking about Omar – what he was up to, and whether he thought about her ever, or why she hadn't turned up to the restaurant that night, and wondering why on earth she'd never been to Italy herself.

January 1991

Although Michael wasn't certain at first that it was his father, he definitely recognised the ruddy-cheeked man in the dirty white Land Rover that was sometimes parked around the corner from school. A black and white collie dog sat beside him in the passenger seat – front paws resting on the window frame – panting in time to the music that was always pouring out of the stereo whenever Michael hurried past.

He was fairly sure it was the same man who had given him that money for his clarinet but it had been such a long time that he couldn't remember the precise features of the man's face, or whether he was just thinking of that photo of his dad, or whether he was getting them altogether mixed up with someone else.

Either way, he sensed the man watching him.

The first time the man spoke to him was one Wednesday, after orchestra, when Michael was in Year Seven. The man greeted him at the end of the road. He was tall and stocky and stood very straight, dressed in jeans and a thick navy fisherman's jumper. And although there was no sign of the car or the dog, Michael knew it was him.

Michael pretended he hadn't heard and headed off purposefully towards the bus stop, rucksack on his back with his clarinet case in one hand and a carrier bag stuffed with sheet music in the other. But the man caught up with him at the traffic lights and tapped him on the shoulder. 'Michael.'

Michael was immediately taken aback by the extreme familiarity of the man's voice – deep and loud and gentle. It reminded him of someone.

'It's me: Dad.' And then he smiled, revealing a dimple in his left cheek that made him look – just for a moment – exactly like John.

Michael flushed. 'Oh, hello.' He started to walk off.

'Wait—'

'I've got to go home, actually. My mum's—'

'Oh, don't worry, I've spoken to Frankie – already explained everything. She wasn't happy about it, if I'm honest.' He pulled a face. 'But she said it's okay, so long as Mike does his homework as soon as he gets in.'

'Oh.' Michael hesitated in the middle of the intersection, glancing at the stream of cars that stretched, unbroken, all the way back to the roundabout.

And so he walked through town with him, this man – his father – who, it transpired, the following week, had bought him a leather music case for his approaching twelfth birthday. But who hadn't wanted, just yet, to buy the pair of wooden clarinets that he had spotted in the classifieds without getting Michael's input first, thinking they could get them together, if he practised hard, gave his old man a hand round the farm from time to time, and did well in his Grade Six.

They sat across the table from one another, that first time, in a cavernous Beefeater pub that sat in a disused car park on the corner of a busy junction just a couple of streets from Michael's home.

It had scaffolding all up the front of the building and it was almost empty inside, except for the barmaid – a middle-aged woman with hair like Cilla Black, a low-cut tee-shirt and a freckly throat – and a couple of men in suits at the bar. They looked up briefly when Michael's father spoke, too loudly, so that Michael shrank back. The barmaid leant in close when she took his order, insisting on bringing their drinks over to the table for them, pretending – the moment they sat down – that she couldn't remember whether Michael's father had ordered lemonade or Coke for his son, just so she had an excuse to come back again.

'It's lemonade for the boy,' Michael's father said – his voice politely firm – but he raised an eyebrow the minute she turned her back. 'They always do that,' he confided.

Michael found it hard to concentrate on what his father was saying, as he watched the way his cigarette smoke hovered like low cloud over their table – conscious of how the smell always clung afterwards to his school blazer, as he sipped his drink, staring at the strange orange glow on the wallpaper just behind his father's head that bounced in time with the repetitive, bleeping, carnival music that screeched from vacant fruit machines.

And that night Michael had one of his dreams.

He woke, not long after he'd fallen asleep, seized with an acute – and total – terror, aware that something evil was in the room with him. His limbs were paralysed. He could not open his eyes. And then a black shape hurtled – flapping and whistling – too close to his face while a tremendous force wrenched him upwards so he felt as though he was being lifted above the bed, hovering beneath the ceiling, looking down on where he'd slept.

And then the light fragmented into shards, colliding, like glass in the end of a kaleidoscope, as he saw himself, dressed all in white, looking out at his father who was standing at the back of a crowd; everyone was watching Michael, clapping and cheering, and he could see his father offering him something. It was a clarinet.

And Michael realised he was being called to play and that was why everyone was there. But just as he reached for the clarinet, he was flung back down to his bed, so hard that he felt a smash in his back as the muscles gave way.

And then he woke up, drenched in sweat.

But he was not in his bed.

He was standing up, the carpet rough and unfamiliar under his feet. And it was so dark that he could not see where the walls were to find the light switch as he shuffled forwards, both arms outstretched, feeling his way towards the edge of the darkness until the fingertips of his right hand brushed the edge of the mattress.

He didn't tell his mum or John that he'd seen his dad. Instead of dropping him off at the front door after that first meeting, his father gave him an awkward goodbye hug and waited at the end of the street, explaining that it wasn't entirely true that he had spoken to Frances. He had *spoken* to her, of course, but he hadn't told her they were meeting that exact day, and he hadn't mentioned anything about the clarinets; she would only disapprove of the cost. 'You know what she's like.'

He felt it should really be their little secret.

So Michael had agreed.

From then on, they met up about once a month – always on a Wednesday – usually going to the same pub – just the two of them. His dad's friend, Andy, a police officer, came along too, a couple of times, if he had a day off – a tall man in pale blue jeans and a tight white shirt tucked in so that his belly hung over his hips as if the shiny leather belt were holding an assembly of body parts together. He lived in Oxford and had been at school with Michael's dad. They weren't really *friends*, as such, his dad had explained, one time when

Michael politely enquired whether Andy would be joining them that day.

'But he's not so bad. We were in a band together once, for about five minutes, when we were a bit older than you. I was on keyboard and vocals and we had *two* bass guitarists for some reason. God knows, we'd have been better off with none. Andy played drums, you see,' his dad always made a point of mentioning whenever the other man was there, 'unusually badly. We were very into the Stones, Fleetwood Mac, Hendrix – all that – but it was a bit beyond us, technically. So we mainly specialised in Doors covers. We were called One Track Mind,' he said solemnly, leaning close so that Michael could smell his soap, like limes. 'Ironic, really, because we did actually only have one track that Andy could manage.' He failed to keep a straight face. 'But what he lacked in talent, he *more* than made up for in determination. Christ, those girls must have kicked themselves.'

Michael smiled back, not wanting to tell his father that he'd told him that story before. Because he loved it when his dad smiled that real smile of his. It seemed to ignite something in the room so that his whole face lit up and his eyes shone, making it impossible to look away.

'Funny your dad doesn't seem to recall his music college phase quite so vividly...' Andy started, one time.

'Oh, leave it.' His dad scraped his chair back and downed his drink.

Andy turned to Michael. 'He'd gone to this audition—'

His father slammed the glass down and stood up. 'Come on then, you,' he said. 'Someone here's got homework to do and those cows won't milk themselves.'

And then, just as suddenly as it had arrived, the smile was gone, like on those first proper days of spring, when the evening comes and everything is cold again, and you forget what it ever meant to feel warm.

He'd taken Michael back to the farm, that April, to show him the new lambs.

'This is the best bit of the year,' he'd explained, swinging the Land Rover into the gravel yard and leading Michael into the farmhouse, chucking him a pair of gigantic black wellingtons from the porch.

As Michael stepped inside the house, he felt an overwhelming sense of déjà vu. The scent from the lavender bush outside the front door carried all the way into the kitchen, lingering somewhere in the distance, with a trace of stale cigarette smoke.

He stopped dead.

An upright piano stood against the back wall alongside a mahogany dresser lined with antique porcelain plates, and as Michael stared, he realised he knew every brush stroke of the raspberry-coloured willow design.

His dad leant against the piano, a cigarette between his teeth as he rooted around in his coat pocket for some matches. 'You alright, Mike?'

Michael nodded and bent down, feeling his fingers tingle as he unlaced his school shoes, knowing exactly how those worn ivory piano keys used to feel under his little palms when he would sit on his dad's knee, on the green velvet piano stool, in an attempt to get them to play, and taken aback by the cold rough flagstones underfoot. The boots were much too big and he stumbled as he tried to stand, grabbing hold of his dad's arm for balance when Gem, the collie, scampered over, planting two wet feet square on Michael's chest.

'I probably shouldn't say this...' His dad shook his head as he strode off across the yard. 'But you're just like your mum sometimes, you know?'

Michael made a face and muttered under his breath as he concentrated on trying to keep up without falling flat in the mud.

The shed was crammed with sheep in small makeshift enclosures and the noise – not to mention the sour smell – was overpowering. His dad pulled open the gate and beckoned to Michael to follow. He leant over the metal railing. 'Come and meet this one.' He grabbed the ewe affectionately, pointing out the red spray-paint on her fleece while the others seemed to all be sprayed in blue. 'This marking's what we do for the twins, you see? She lambed this morning.' He crouched down.

Michael noticed two tiny black and white speckled creatures that looked more like Dalmatian puppies than lambs, sheltering under their mother.

'Can you see? They've got the same red marks as mum in case they get split up. This little one's my favourite.' His father pulled the ewe back by the scruff of the neck so she was facing them again. He looked the animal straight in the eye. 'I'm just going to have a quick hold, okay?'

He reached down and lifted up one of the lambs, cradling it very gently in his arms. Its face was narrow and too long for its body with a patch of scruffy wool between the eyes, like an old-fashioned teddy bear. It made no struggle. 'I'm too soft for this nonsense, Mike.' He laughed. 'Rule number one: never get attached to anything you're going to have to get shot of.'

He twisted the neck of the lamb towards Michael.

'But just look at that face, won't you?'

The lamb watched Michael – its small black eyes constantly checking all around while the head never moved.

'This is the meat of it,' his father said, in such a soft voice that Michael almost missed it. 'You never get tired of this stuff. Trust me.' He patted the ewe to soothe her. And then he stood up and gestured to Michael. 'Ready? Your turn now.' He carefully delivered the animal into Michael's arms, but the minute he stepped back, the lamb let out a screech and struggled, writhing, suddenly incredibly heavy as Michael's father let go – bony limbs kicking in all directions and enormous up close, while its mother – bleating loudly – bashed the crown of her head against the side of the fence, so that Michael shouted out in distress for his dad to take it off him.

And when Michael looked up at his dad, he was taken aback by the expression of total calm in his eyes as he stood, very still, soothing the lamb and the ewe until they had both stopped crying.

Back in the farmhouse, after he had shown Michael the side barn where the different feeds were stored and the special trick with the lids to stop the rats getting in, his dad sat him down at the kitchen table and insisted on showing him the shotgun – how to hold it properly, how the safety mechanism worked, but most important of all, how to make sure the cabinet was properly locked – from both sides – and where to always make sure you put the keys.

'Because a farmer's boy's got to know these things. It's irresponsible not to.' He sat down, laying the case on the table between them.

Michael had felt his whole body tighten the moment his father unlocked the cabinet.

'Who knows?' said his dad, clicking open the case. 'One of these days it'll be you sitting here with your boy.'

Michael shook his head. He stood up too quickly, knocking his chair over as he backed away towards the wall.

'It's alright, Mike. I'm not going to—'

'I don't like it.' He could feel his teeth chattering. He couldn't take his eyes off the shiny black metal. He felt his face hurting, as if he were about to cry.

'Hey, it's okay. I'm putting it away now. I'll show you another time.'

His dad locked the cabinet and put the keys in a drawer.

But Michael couldn't move.

'Come back.' His father dragged one of the kitchen chairs over to the piano and sat down. 'Help me out with the right hand, will you?'

He patted the stool beside him and after a while, when Michael still hadn't moved, his dad started to play. He didn't once look down at his hands, and although the sheet music was tucked behind another piece on the stand, Michael immediately recognised the melancholic opening bars of the nocturne that he had been practising for his exam.

His dad didn't talk to Michael so much when Andy was there and Andy rarely spoke to Michael directly except to ask about his mother.

'She was a bit of a looker, your mum,' Andy had said, with a teasing smile, the first time Michael met him, his hairy fingers clasped around his Guinness, tapping his signet ring against the glass. Michel noticed the way the foam always caught on his top lip. 'What's she up to these days?'

'I don't know, really.' Michael stared at the tabletop, his palms sweaty against the cool glass, as his father listened on, in rigid silence, before pretending to laugh along.

'Bit long in the tooth now, eh, Mike?' He ruffled Michael's hair too hard.

Michael shrugged.

He hated it when his father called him Mike.

It sounded as though he was talking about somebody else's son.

'Coming up to forty now, isn't she?' His father watched him, waiting for him to agree – to nod or laugh along – anything at all to show whose side he was on – while Andy just sat there, his eyes, above the rim of the glass, never once shifting from Michael's father.

'It's her birthday on Monday. She'll be thirty-eight,' Michael said, looking down and sipping his drink, picturing his mother seen from his bedroom window, down in the garden – kneeling – as she bedded in the new magnolia shrub that he and John had helped her choose from the garden centre for her birthday.

It was drizzling. The knees of her jeans were soaked through and stained with green, her long angular face frowning in concentration as she patted down the earth with her giant, rough gardening gloves, her fine dark hair, streaked now with tiny strands of grey, tied back in a faded blue headscarf to keep it out of her all-seeing, quiet brown eyes – worried, on those Wednesdays when she got home before him to find that he was not back from school yet. He used to look away when he told her that orchestra had overrun again so he didn't have to see the concern in those eyes – the kindest eyes ever to have been planted in a human face.

August 1998

In the end it was an advert in the Sunday travel supplement that swung it. They were advertising last-minute all-inclusive week-long holidays to Chania, on the north-west coast of Crete. They only needed two pictures to persuade her: one of a tiny shingle beach – sea the colour of petrol – with no-one in sight, and another that took her down a cobbled street, a church at one end, with an elderly man in a cap, squatting on the quay, dragging in a giant fishing net.

She picked up the phone and booked it there and then.

She hadn't mentioned to John and Olivia that she was thinking of going away. But when the tickets arrived the following week, she left them propped against the fruit bowl so that John asked her about it the minute he got home from work.

'Oh, I just fancied a bit of a change of scene, I guess,' she explained, glancing up from the cryptic crossword, as her son busied himself with what appeared to be the complicated lemon and caper risotto recipe that Susanna Whitaker had painstakingly described to Frankie, on two separate occasions during her first week in hospital, having wrestled it from the chef in the restaurant they'd specifically returned to in Il Campo – '*hang* the expense, as Brian put it; it's not every day that your only daughter gets engaged' – on their last day in Siena.

June 1991

'He's gifted, your son.'

Mrs Barrington – Michael's form teacher – had intercepted Frankie at the door of the brightly lit school sports hall the moment Frankie had arrived – late and on edge – at the Year Seven parents' evening, one Monday towards the start of the second half of the summer term, and sat her down, briefly, to prepare her for the comments that would follow from Michael's teachers.

The hall was packed; she looked around, nodding politely in the direction of a few faces that looked vaguely familiar – never entirely sure if she recognised them from the surgery or the school. The noise echoed off the walls that were stacked high with gymnastics equipment – rubber mats, benches and vaulting boxes that were chained to the ceiling to prevent everything from falling.

Frankie was finding it hard to tune into the teacher's voice above the din. She had been working extra shifts to pay her dad back the final instalment of the loan for the house and she'd struggled to get there for half-past six. Although she knew it was unlikely, she was worried Callum might turn up, like that time five years earlier when John started at the school. She kept an eye on the door just in case and politely declined when the teacher offered her a cup of tea or coffee, gesturing to the people queuing at Formica folding tables at the back.

She steeled herself as she approached the music teacher who had been watching her from the other side of the room since she arrived – a thin, frail-looking young woman. She couldn't have been more than twenty-five or so but something about the way she wore her hair – in a limp white-blonde ponytail, parted heavily down the centre so that the two bangs drooped low on either side – made her look twice her age. She had a serious expression that seemed to disapprove of all that she beheld through those spectacles with the sort of transparent frames that camouflaged into her face which, with its puddingy pink cheeks and watery blue eyes, would perhaps have benefited from a touch more concealment. So this was her: Miss Albany, the woman that Michael talked about every evening with a reverence that Frankie found disturbing.

Miss Albany stood up, smoothing her long paisley skirt. She clasped Frankie's hands to hers. 'Mrs Webb – it must be,' she said, lisping a little, as if she had recently started wearing an orthodontic brace. 'I can see the likeness immediately.'

Frankie's smile was tight-lipped. 'It's nice to meet you, Miss Albany.' She sat down on the brown plastic chair and tried not to roll her programme too conspicuously in her hands.

The young woman put down her papers. 'Where to begin?' She threw her hands up. 'Michael. What a joy to teach,' she declared – her voice nasal as if those spectacles pinched, rather. 'I've never had a student so dedicated, so determined to learn. He's nearly there, you know, with the circular breathing.'

'Right,' said Frankie cautiously.

'And you know he's started teaching himself the piano? In the lunchbreak. Did you know that, Mrs Webb?' she said, a look of glee in her eyes.

Frankie had a sudden memory of Callum, at the piano, after Christmas – Michael's first.

Miss Albany was staring at her.

'I didn't know that. That's… wonderful.'

'He's ever so modest, though, isn't he? Whenever any of us praises him, he says – in that *way* of his – "It's not me, it's my talent". She laughed in delight.

Frankie stared straight ahead.

'He's more of a teaching assistant than a pupil, to be honest.' She laughed again – a braying sound that was unnaturally loud.

Frankie tried to smile back. But her face was aching.

'I'd strongly suggest that he be encouraged to join as many extracurricular groups as possible – wind bands… local youth orchestras – you name it. And we'll continue to go out of our way to make sure he explores all the instruments he likes, here, during the school day. For it would be *criminal* to let a talent like that go unnourished.' She raised an eyebrow.

Frankie stiffened. 'Of… of course,' she stammered. 'We've already looked into it – Michael and I; he's been playing in the church group for a while now but there's a Saturday morning thing, too – very close to us. We were thinking of starting him over the holidays.'

The teacher was nodding very seriously, a look of concern on her face. 'Yes, it is an absolute must, Mrs Webb. I can't stress it strongly enough. You have a very gifted son,' she declared.

Again, that word. Why did they all say it in that peculiar voice?

Frankie glanced at the door again, accidentally catching Mrs Barrington's eye. She was watching her. Frankie dutifully waved her programme as she quickly looked back down. She still had nine other appointments and she needed to be getting back to the boys.

'I look forward to seeing you at the concert,' Miss Albany said, standing up to shake Frankie's hand when the ten minutes were up.

'Concert?' Frankie was worried now that she wasn't going to get home in time. She needed to take her jacket off. Her face felt very hot.

'Yes. It's the last week of term; we're doing a special *Carmen* arrangement. But Michael also has a solo. Hasn't he mentioned it?' She leant towards Frankie in confidence. 'He's chosen the Poulenc – the second movement.'

'Has he?' Frankie said, feeling her face tremble as a funny pain started to seep upwards from her stomach. 'His dad's favourite...' Her fingers began to tingle.

There was a sudden metallic taste in her mouth and she coughed. She flexed her hands, sensing the tiny grey speckles start to crowd in on her vision.

'I told him I thought it was too demanding,' the teacher brayed, 'but he insisted.' She was staring at Frankie. 'Are you alright, Mrs Webb?'

Frankie's stomach felt heavy. And she was breathing too fast. She tried to nod.

'You must be very proud.'

Frankie battled with the top button of her jacket. It took all her concentration. 'Is it just me or is it hot in here?' She was aware that her voice sounded too deep. 'Yes, we're extremely proud. Of course, I'll be there.' Saliva filled her mouth and she tried to breathe more slowly, through her nose. 'Thank you,' she added, attempting to smile, before heading blindly towards the door.

When she asked Michael about the concert later that evening, he looked surprised.

'Oh, that,' he said. 'It's no big deal. I thought I'd mentioned it, actually. Sure – come if you want,' he added doubtfully. 'I *think* parents are invited.'

She hesitated. 'Okay,' she said. 'In that case, I'd love to.'

*

But the night before the concert Michael had seemed particularly withdrawn. Orchestra rehearsal had gone on even later than normal and when he came in, he told her that he had already had something to eat. And then he had gone straight up to his room.

She'd gone to bed herself not long afterwards and read for a while but couldn't concentrate, so switched off the light and tried to get some sleep. Down the street someone had left a gate open and it was knocking in the wind.

As she started to breathe slowly out, something smashed down on her face.

She screamed.

Her top lip was crushed against her front teeth, which grazed the damp palm of a hand.

She smelt appley shampoo.

'Michael!' she gasped. 'Get off me.'

'Mum!' He was sobbing.

She struggled against the weight of him.

'Where am I?' He let out a shrill wail. 'Where are you?'

She hauled herself up and switched on the light.

He was cowering by the bed. 'I had a bad dream.'

She breathed out loudly and held him close. 'It's okay, it's me. It's just a dream.'

He cupped his hands over his ears. 'It's that voice. I can't get rid of it.'

She said nothing, simply stayed there, stroking his hair, until he was calm. And then, when her heartbeat had returned almost to normal, she led him back to his bed.

She decided not to go to the concert in the end. She wasn't sure she could face it. She hadn't been able to sleep after putting Michael back to bed and made up her mind to book an appointment, first thing the next morning, with her GP, Dr Carmichael, to talk about the anxiety. Privately, she was worried that the music might upset her, too, and she didn't want to go to pieces in front of all those people.

Besides, Michael had seemed so reluctant for her to come when she brought it up again that morning. He said he thought it might put him off – and anyhow, he'd heard that someone would probably be filming it, so they could just get a copy of the video afterwards.

But John went. He had to, he explained when they got home that evening, his face haggard, after Michael had gone up to put his clarinet away.

'It was a massive deal, Mum. Michael was totally downplaying it but all the teachers were talking about it all day and everything.' He reached for the bottle of flat cola that Frankie kept at the back of the cupboard to keep the nausea at bay. The label had come unstuck so it clung like a loose sleeve around the flabby plastic, and although she started to protest as he lifted it straight to his lips, he looked so unsettled that she stopped herself.

She sat down. His expression reminded her of something that had happened a long time before and she wondered if he remembered anything of that particular day. But she knew she could never ask him.

'It was the way he was standing before he did his solo. Like a statue, with his arms behind his back. He had put his clarinet on that little stand on the floor in front of him. And he was all in white, for some reason, even though everyone else was just in normal uniform.'

Frankie clasped her hands tightly around her knee. She nodded, gently encouraging him to go on.

'He had his eyes closed. As though he was concentrating really hard. Some kids in Year Eleven were laughing but I don't think he heard. And then when he started playing, he swayed to the music, like this,' he said, demonstrating. 'As if he was a professional musician or something. It was *so* embarrassing.' He shook his head.

Frankie smiled and raised her eyebrows. 'Right.' She tried to control the tremble at the corners of her mouth. 'Is that it?' she said, foolishly hopeful.

'Oh my God, no.' He rolled his eyes. 'After he'd finished, everyone was clapping – he *is* really good, you know. Dominic's mum kept going on about how good he was afterwards.' John took another swig.

Frankie waited, as if cemented to her seat. And for once, when he belched, she didn't say anything.

'So then he goes off down the side of the stage; everyone obviously thinks he's finished but instead of sitting down with everyone else, he goes up to the music teacher – she was doing all the piano stuff – and then he…' John trailed off.

'Yes?' Frankie waited – her eyes hot and too dry.

'I think he was trying to shake her hand or pat her on the back or something but he accidentally sort of fell on her.'

'What?' She stood up, hand over her mouth. 'What did she do?'

He tried to suppress a horrified smile. 'She was really surprised, *obviously*, and she sort of pushed him away – politely – but really quite hard – and then he went and sat down. But he had this really odd look on his face – a weird smile.'

John looked away.

Frankie stared straight ahead.

'And then there was the other thing,' he said, his voice quieter now, as if unsure of himself now, and he glanced over nervously, to check her reaction.

'What else?' Frankie's voice had dropped. She tried to breathe more deeply.

'Well, he'd obviously asked Dad to come.'

Frankie sat down, hard.

The light was too bright behind John.

Frankie felt a darkness start to push, from the edge of her eyes, across her vision as the pins and needles started in her hands. She reached for the bottle John was holding and tried to raise it to her lips but it was too heavy. She couldn't swallow.

'He was really late,' she heard him say. 'It was definitely him. He must have just meant to get there in time for Michael's bit. I saw Michael waving to him when he sat down. I kept my head down but when he saw me, he kept looking over. I think he thought you might have been there.'

'Did he…?' Frankie started but there wasn't enough air in her throat and she thought she was going to be sick.

'No, he didn't speak to me, thank goodness – not that I'd have spoken to him even if he did. I'm not a complete idiot. I just went out the other way afterwards, so I didn't have to go past him.' He frowned. 'But they were chatting for ages in the playground and he gave Michael this massive hug. I saw him. By the gate.' He paused. 'They've obviously been hanging out a bit.'

Frankie didn't say anything. The light was unbearable now.

And then came a voice from nowhere.

'Why are you always talking about me?'

In the background, a dark shape filled the doorway. It looked like Callum. But it must have been Michael.

She tried to get up but felt she might fall over.

And she wondered how long he had been standing there.

'Help me, John,' she growled. 'I feel a bit funny. I need to lie down.'

John held her around the waist and guided her, past Michael, up the stairs.

Frankie lay on the bed until the feelings had passed and her vision had returned to normal. And then she went back downstairs to rejoin her sons who were chatting in front of the television, as if nothing had happened. She could tell from the bleeping that John was playing Tetris.

She stood in the doorway. The news was on. She sat down between them and they fell, one by one, into silence as they watched a report on the ongoing BSE crisis following the latest outbreak – on a farm in Surrey. The reporter, who was standing in a stable-yard beside a farmer waiting to be interviewed, paused while a voiceover explained the impact on British beef exports – a line-graph hovering over a blurry photograph of slaughtered cattle – as the camera zoomed in on a dead calf, so young that its hooves hadn't even been trimmed, before cutting back to the reporter.

Frankie bit her lip, trying not to picture Callum, alone, at the kitchen table in the farmhouse while in the background, a girl led two horses across the screen.

And then came scenes of total devastation following the cyclone in Bangladesh a few weeks earlier. Whole villages were still submerged in water and rubble, and trees were still blocking access to recovery efforts. Above the sound of wailing, men waded – waist-deep – to retrieve their families and their livelihoods in a wasteland that had once been a home.

Michael shook his head in horror and turned to her with tears in his eyes. 'Mum,' he said. 'How can this happen?'

She lay a hand on his shoulder, forgetting just then about all the other things. 'He'd have been so proud, your dad,' she whispered.

*

She would telephone the school the very next day to apologise to Miss Albany on behalf of her son. And the teachers would unanimously agree, with great generosity, to excuse the entire affair, understanding it to be one of Michael's little eccentricities – seeing, all too clearly, that he had simply been caught up with the excitement of the evening. They would insist she think no more about it and reassure her that it had been a wonderful concert and that Michael's performance in particular had been nothing short of extraordinary.

But when she picked up the newspaper to sit down alongside her children that evening, Frankie found that she could not think of a single thing to say to them. Instead, she pretended that nothing had changed as she sat in silence, as if in deep concentration. She stared so long at the crossword that the little black and white squares started to dance in front of one another, blurring the outlines of the evening, like so many before and since, giving way eventually to a big black hole where a family should have been.

August 1998

'So, Liv thinks you don't like her parents,' John said, in a matter-of-fact tone, as he served up the risotto.

'What?' Frankie flushed.

'Or her.'

'What do you mean? I love Olivia. And her parents.'

He deliberately avoided her gaze. 'She thinks you think she's not good enough and that's why you don't want to go on that spa thing with her and her mum.'

Frankie laughed. 'That's ridiculous. It's got nothing to do with it. It's two hundred and fifty pounds, John. You know I haven't got that kind of money.'

'Brian's paying. She already said that.'

Frankie shook her head. 'I don't want him to pay for me. I just can't justify spending all that money on… It's not right.'

'It's not about you, Mum. It's Liv's day. If she wants it, then why—'

'No, I'm sure we could find something just as nice. I'll look into it. Don't worry.'

He was quiet for a while. 'It's not just that.' He looked her in the eye. '*I don't think you like her either.*'

She reached for his hand. 'I don't know her that well,' she ventured. 'I probably don't understand her entirely yet.'

'What's that supposed to mean?'

'Come on, John. You're the one getting married to her. Do *you* love her? That's what matters.'

'Yes, I think so,' he said unhappily. 'She's great. She's just *normal* – you know – gorgeous, obviously – everyone says so...'

Frankie pulled a face. 'She's not a doll, John.'

'I didn't mean that,' he snapped. 'Why do you twist everything?'

'Sorry.' Frankie sipped her wine.

'She always knows what to do. She's organised – good at sorting things. Do you know what I mean?'

Frankie nodded doubtfully. 'And do you want the same things, do you think, for the future? Trust me – marriage isn't all lavender bags and smoked salmon vol au vents. It's damned hard work.'

'It can't be *that* hard,' he retorted, rolling his eyes. 'Most people manage it, don't they?'

She flinched.

'I thought you'd be happy for me.'

'I am happy for you,' she said evenly, trying not to bite her lip.

They ate in silence for a while.

'What I'm trying to say, I think, is: do you see eye to eye on the big things? Have you talked about – I don't know – children – money – work – what you want to *do* – where you want to *be*?'

'I guess so. But we haven't talked about that sort of stuff out loud exactly. She's quite caught up with all her LPC stuff at the moment. And I just sort of assumed she'd probably want the same things as me.'

'And what *is* that, exactly, John?' she pressed gently.

'I don't know. Kids and stuff. Just a normal family.'

Frankie sat back and concentrated on her food. 'Right,' she said, reaching over and squeezing his hand, hoping he didn't see her expression. It reminded her of a conversation she had had years before with Michael.

But she thought about what John had said.

And when they had finished, she looked at him directly. 'I think that's probably what I always wanted as well.' She smiled. 'A normal family. But I wouldn't wonder if the normal ones are pretty weird too, on the whole.' She attempted a laugh. 'You know, from the inside, looking out.'

July 1991

In the weeks that followed the concert Frankie asked Michael, more than once, whether he had heard from his father lately.

'Oh, you know, now and then,' Michael would say, rarely looking up from his books. 'Occasionally he pops by to see me at the school gate but I don't see him much, really. I mean, he's family, isn't he? But I hardly know him, Mum,' he said to her once, looking right at her, an expression of curiosity on his lips. 'Do I?'

But she didn't believe him. She couldn't tell if she was imagining it but she thought she sensed something teasing – cryptic – whenever he mentioned his father, almost as if he knew the effect it had on her. And so, instead, she just pretended to believe him, and brushed the remarks away, as with all their other little opportunities for anything that might have passed, in any other home, for intimacy.

No, eventually things got back to normal and it wasn't until two or three years later, in fact, when John started to bring back little nuggets of worry again, here and there, that Frankie was forced to pay more attention to the unmistakable changes in Michael's demeanour. She couldn't pretend any longer, even to herself, that things were anywhere near alright. Never more so than when Michael told her, one evening at the end of the summer term, that he'd prefer to start calling her Frances.

'What?' She laughed, accidentally knocking her cup of tea so that it wobbled and splashed on an old pile of *Hello!*

magazines from the surgery. 'Why?' she snapped, grabbing a cloth.

'It feels more respectful.'

'Oh, no, I don't think so. You sound like my mother.' She pushed the cloth hard into the laughing face of Princess Diana, already soaked through from the log ride.

'No,' she said again, staring at the frozen expression on the face of her son.

She'd ripped a hole right through it.

'You're not to call me that. It's weird. I don't like it.'

But he seemed to have made up his mind.

She was dreading the day when John went to university, leaving her alone with Michael. What would they talk about? There was something about the way he had looked at John's new girlfriend, Olivia, when she and a couple of others had popped round one evening on the last day of term. It had reminded her of Callum – just a shred of lasciviousness in his smile that she could never be sure, entirely, that she hadn't imagined.

The change unsettled her.

For in every other respect Michael maintained a persona that seemed entirely asexual – prudish – to the extent of appearing a little disapproving even – when he saw people kiss on the street. And she pretended not to notice when he shielded his gaze from the occasional moment of forced intimacy when they watched TV together.

Because she didn't like to admit that she was glad he did.

One Christmas, during *Songs of Praise*, he had asked her what a virgin was. She had blushed and got up from the sofa, to turn up the volume.

'It's a... an unmarried woman,' she had muttered.

'Are you a virgin, then?' he said.

She bristled, her back, still, to her son. 'No, Michael, because I've been married before – to your dad. You know that.'

'You mean you're a celibate, then?' he said solemnly.

'No,' she snapped, reaching blindly for a book that had been left on the floor. 'I'm not celibate. I'm...' she hesitated, 'I'm... separated.'

She could feel his eyes on her as she leafed through John's copy of *Far from the Madding Crowd*. It was stuffed full of little yellow Post-it notes and he had underlined every other word in wobbly blue biro.

'Like me,' he said.

'What?' She spun around.

He was nodding but his mouth looked uncertain – worried. 'I'm separated from my father, too, aren't I, Frances?'

'No,' she said too quickly, looking back down at the book. 'That's different.'

'Not in his eyes, it's not,' he said, his voice barely audible now.

She sat back down, pitching one elbow on the arm of the sofa and cradling her cheek in her hand. 'Whose eyes?' she whispered.

'My father's.'

Her face felt warm, as if she had been sitting by the fire.

'Why *are* we all separated, Frances? Is it because of me?'

'No.' She shook her head. 'Of course not.'

'Then why can't we all be a proper family? Why are we all alone?'

She stared at him. 'We *are* a proper family. We love you very much. It's just that it wasn't right for us all to stay together because...' She faltered.

Michael looked down at his hands. 'Why did you have to break up our family?' he whispered.

'I didn't,' she pleaded. 'It wasn't like that. It was just the situation – it was all too much – with the farm – and the…' She trailed off. 'He's not a happy man, Michael, your dad. I couldn't be who he wanted me to be.'

Michael wiped away a tear.

He looked her bravely in the eye. 'Are *you* a happy person, then?'

The question caught her by surprise.

'Did you become what you wanted to be?'

'No, yes, of course.' She spluttered. 'I don't know what I wanted to be. I wanted to be a mum, I suppose.'

It was a while before he spoke.

'No-one's happy all the time.'

'No, I know – of course not. But there's happiness and there's *happiness*, isn't there?' She thought about what she was trying to say, aware that it probably made no sense. 'And I don't think he wanted me to be *allowed* to be the person I wanted to be either, if you follow? I think he was angry he couldn't be what *he* wanted to be.'

She realised she had never said any of this out loud to anyone. And she remembered that thing Callum used to say: 'The shitty stuff in life – that's the meat of it; you can't just walk away from it.'

And it was as if she were seeing it all clearly now for the first time, laid out in front of her, as if that's how things had always been, set – still – rather than how it had all felt at the time, like a complex jigsaw puzzle that she was caught in the middle of, trying to climb out, but unsure what went where and with all the corner pieces missing.

'He never wanted the farm either, Michael, not really, but if you'd met *his* father… now there's a difficult man, to put it mildly.' She raised her eyebrows. 'With – let's just say – some very fixed ideas of what everyone else – your dad in particular – should do. He should have been a musician, your dad, like you.'

'Oh.' Michael looked away.

'And some people can't be happy because they can't be their real self. They're trapped – always trying to be someone else – someone that they think everyone else thinks they should be.'

They sat in silence for a while.

'But isn't that silly, Michael?' She reached for his hand. 'We only have one life. What's the point of wasting that precious gift, pretending to be something we're not?'

'I think he just needed someone to help him,' Michael said quietly.

'Well, who doesn't?' she retorted. 'Besides, there are plenty of people who can help him.'

Michael didn't say anything.

'He knew it would be like that.' She shook her head. 'He can't say no-one warned him. It's the nature of the beast. He knew it. He used to say, "No-one's in it for the money; there's never any money. You've got to do it for the sheer love of it."'

She paused.

'Like a lot of jobs,' he said.

She stared at him.

'Or maybe just because otherwise it won't survive,' she said eventually.

He sat so still that she wasn't sure if he'd even heard her. And then he stood up.

'It's okay, Frances. Don't worry,' he whispered, leaning over her to kiss her goodnight. 'He'll forgive you if you say sorry.'

She didn't say anything. Her eyes were too hot, now, for their sockets.

But she had an awful dream that night. She was back on the farm; a pigeon had got into the kitchen and she couldn't

Scenes from Childhood

get it out. It flapped around her face, screeching like a child, as she waved it outside. And even though the door was unlocked, she had no strength, so that however hard she pushed, it would not budge. And when the door finally gave way, the screaming stopped. And she pushed the bird too firmly, realising too late that it was Michael, just as it crashed against the frame of the door, falling at her feet.

September 1998

As the weeks passed and the departure date duly approached, Frankie sensed a tingle of her old nerves creeping back. She'd never been on holiday on her own before. And it occurred to her that she hadn't been abroad since her honeymoon, and that was over twenty years ago, she realised, with a pang of longing, as she tried not to think about the girl she had been back then or that photograph that Callum had sent her – so young and pretty and carefree – and picturing herself now, all alone, in a restaurant, in the midst of all the other normal families on their holidays, fretting about what on earth she was going to wear.

But it was the flight that was really worrying her. It was over four hours. And she wasn't sure she was going to be able to cope.

In the end, two days before she was due to travel, she rang Dr Carmichael and booked an emergency appointment, 'for vaccinations', explaining somewhat cagily to Debbie, the other receptionist, who was delighted to hear from her, that she was going 'abroad' for a little while but would certainly drop in to the surgery to see them all when she got back.

He had kindly offered to give her a telephone appointment first thing the next morning and agreed reluctantly, when she finally came clean about the purpose of her call, to prescribe a very brief course of Valium – 'but only for the flight'. One tablet to test at home that night in case of any reaction, and two more – one each way – for the journey. She could collect it from her local pharmacy – he'd fax it over.

July 1994

Although it was hard to pinpoint what had changed, exactly, in Michael – or when – she recalled one particular evening that stood out.

It must have been the summer just before John started at Warwick University because they'd spent the day together, she and John, at IKEA, getting some bits for his room in halls. She hadn't slept well the previous night and had been secretly dreading the trip to Croydon.

But she had been surprised by what a lovely time they had ended up having. And had been delighted when John had casually suggested, after Frankie had finally agreed to the chrome CD rack, despite the wooden one being just as nice and almost four pounds cheaper, that maybe Olivia might like to come round for dinner the following evening. Frankie had been pestering him for weeks to invite her over so that she and Michael could get to know her a bit better; yes, of course she remembered chatting to her after that rugby match, but you could hardly classify that as 'getting to know' someone, could you? And it was important. Especially now she and John were thinking of going on holiday together.

On top of that, they'd managed to go the whole day without mentioning Michael once. So, it caught her somewhat off-guard when John asked her – when they got home, after dinner – whether she thought there was something up with Michael.

She couldn't remember where Michael had been at the time

– he must have been out at church or down at the homeless shelter in St Ebbes, possibly; he'd recently started volunteering there as part of his Duke of Edinburgh award; Monira, the woman who ran it, was the mum of a girl at the school. But when John said that, she had a sudden image of Michael, from the previous night, crouched over his Bible. She had been calling him but he hadn't heard, and when he finally noticed her in the doorway, there was a wild expression in his eyes and his mouth was ferocious. His face immediately dropped when he saw her but he had smiled too quickly, and the smile hadn't matched the eyes. 'Hello, Frances,' he had said.

'What do you mean by strange?' she had said to John a little sharply, standing up too quickly to clear away the plates. She sniffed, puzzled, and checked the cooker a second time, twisting the knobs all the way around and back again, twice, to make sure it was certainly switched off. 'John, can you smell gas?'

'Mum.' He rolled his eyes. 'That's the third time you've asked me that. Honestly, there's no smell.'

'Sorry – go on.'

'I don't know. He's been spending so much time with the church lot. And did you know he's stopped going to orchestra?'

She stared at him and shook her head.

All she could see was Michael, the night before – that strange guttural sound and the elastic movement of his mouth. 'I'd prefer it if you knocked, Frances,' he'd said.

When she'd asked him what language he'd been speaking, he had turned away, sliding the book beneath his bed.

'Mum, are you even listening?'

Frankie stared blankly at him. 'Sorry, John. What did you say?'

'I thought that was odd.' John's mouth twisted. 'But when I

asked him about it, he said he didn't think it was right to just play while there was so much suffering.'

The words hung between them.

Frankie's insides felt cold and she forced a brittle laugh. 'Did he? Oh, he's always been a bit of an oddball, hasn't he?' She reached over to hug her son around the shoulder.

But John stiffened and moved away.

'Olivia said one of her friends had seen him with Leighton Harrison by the canal. You know that really weird goth kid in Year Ten who's got a snake?'

She winced. 'Well, it's no good you worrying—'

John threw his arms up. 'Why can't you *do* something?'

'What do you mean?' She turned away to make a start on the dishes. 'Come on, John,' she said firmly. 'Michael's just Michael. He's fine. He's just going through a bit of a spiritual phase at the moment.' She stared blindly at her reflection in the kitchen window. 'Leave him alone. He'll grow out of it.'

John was silent for a while but when he spoke again there was an accusatory tone to his voice that she didn't recognise. 'He's obviously not fine. Why do you keep pretending?'

Her face burnt.

'You know, you can be a really crap mum sometimes.'

She froze.

'Maybe,' she said eventually, her voice unrecognisably low.

In the reflection, she saw him drop his head. 'Sorry, Mum.' He sniffed. 'I didn't mean that. I just wish someone else could deal with all his shit sometimes.'

Her mouth moved but no sound came out. She cleared her throat. 'I can't talk about this right now,' she whispered, turning away to get rid of the ghastly face of her own mother, contorted in sorrow, staring back at her through the same wild eyes. 'I'll have a think. And in the meantime, if he's being a bit weird, well, just try to ignore it for now. At least it's not drugs or knives or something.' She tried to laugh, pulling the plug, watching the contaminated water draining noisily away, but her throat was too tight and the air got stuck. She turned the tap again, squirting in more soap.

John's voice was subdued. 'I miss the old Michael a bit.'

They were silent for a while, weighing the words between them.

'I hope he doesn't go and do anything stupid.'

She nodded. 'Don't worry about him,' she said, sponging and sponging the same plate. Her voice no longer belonged to her. And the water was too hot, turning her hands a deep purple – the plate so clean that it made a scraping sound, blunted only by the bubbles.

She wanted to hold her son close, wishing beyond anything that she could have faith in her own foolish words. But she couldn't even look him in the eye. 'Everything will be fine,' she had added, staring instead at the lying mouth of the woman opposite her in the glass, realising, as her son withdrew to the darkness, that she no longer knew her.

***

It meant that Frankie was perpetually prepared, though – or on her guard – as she tried to describe that feeling of anxiety to the GP, that kept her from sleeping for night after night – or 'a state of hyper-vigilance', as Dr Carmichael had suggested helpfully, looking something up in his book as he sifted through family histories for medicinal remedies.

'As if one were awaiting an announcement of some description, perhaps? Or at least a significant change?'

But all the while Frankie kept telling herself that there was no point fighting the inevitable. Whatever was to come, she would find a way to cope because, after all, she reasoned, her worst fear had already been confirmed long ago. She knew Michael and Callum were still in touch. And she had coped with that, hadn't she?

Well, sort of, she reflected, recalling that strange phone call she'd received, not long after she'd got back from work one evening, when Michael was out at the homeless shelter.

The person hadn't said anything when she picked up.

But she'd heard what sounded like a piano playing in the background – and then a man's voice, muffled, while someone else breathed, too calmly, in the mouthpiece.

And it made her wonder, sometimes, whether he really was going to church, or helping Monira out at the homeless shelter, as he said he was, or whether he was, in fact, spending some of the time with his father.

And although she did her best to put the thoughts out of her mind, trying her hardest to convince herself that all of that would just go away when Michael did, she nevertheless watched her youngest with a curious intensity.

Typically, when Michael chose to reveal his hand, one Monday evening in late November, he timed it perfectly to coincide with the one time in the week that she reserved exclusively for herself, to be pleasantly distracted for an entire thirty minutes during *Panorama*.

It had only just started; he must have heard the music from upstairs and he came in and sat down right next to her on the arm of the sofa.

He had not long got back from church and she rather pointedly turned the volume up as she reluctantly shuffled along to make room for him.

She showed no surprise when he observed aloud that he

had been thinking about the future, explaining that they had been going through A-Level options again at school that day.

'I know it's a long way off but it got me thinking about university and jobs and all that. I thought it might be good to take some time off before starting university – travel a bit – across Europe, maybe; South America.'

Although she was waiting, like a cat, to pounce on the slightest bit of further information, she had simply nodded casually, as if only half-listening – trying not to look too positive too soon.

'I know it's expensive, before you say anything, but I had a word with the guy who runs that new sandwich shop on the High Street. He needs someone on Saturdays, apparently. We could save up.'

She hadn't looked directly at him but in the reflection of the television screen she had watched him – this serious young man, perched there, still in his grey school uniform trousers and a cream and brown striped collarless woven shirt, with his brown bootlace necklace to which he had recently suspended a small wooden cross. He had cut his hair much shorter recently and it suited him, disarming her, every time she saw him, by how much he resembled Callum when she had first met him. It was something about the look in his eyes – a newly discovered defiance – that had emerged as if overnight. And she found herself wondering – albeit doubtfully – whether perhaps he had met someone.

He wasn't sure exactly where he'd go yet. 'Except Rome, obviously, and Greece.' He paused. 'And Spain, too, probably.'

'A sort of Interrailing thing, then?' she had said hopefully. 'Like John and Olivia did?'

'Sort of...' he had conceded.

As she watched him, quietly sipping his peppermint tea,

she had a sudden glimpse into the future; her youngest son, on the cusp of leaving home. She felt a wrench of panic. It was too late. That day would be upon her before she knew it. And he would be gone.

She saw in a flash the few short years that remained – stretching out in front of her, like an empty room with no window. And she reached out for him, clutching his arm so tightly that he had to pass the cup to the other hand to avoid spilling it.

'Maybe I could come out for a long weekend or something to see you?' She smiled uncertainly. 'I've always wanted to visit Rome.'

He looked puzzled and patted her awkwardly. 'I see,' he said with a smile.

And as he talked about his travels Frankie felt a surge of unexpected pride in him. He was destined for great things, this young man. He was special. And she realised, only after Michael had left the room, that *Panorama* was finished. She hadn't heard a single thing, not even the introduction, and now she had missed it entirely. And yet instead of disappointment she felt the beginnings of a warm release, seeing the years open up in front of her, like a door flung wide on to a new future.

For he would be gone not just for that whole summer but likely six or seven months. The more he had talked, the more apparent it became that he had an extremely lucid and well-planned itinerary in front of him. More than that – he had never been clearer in his mind about exactly what it was that he wanted.

She had nodded, listening, and had said very little but gradually felt herself coming around to the idea. For although she would miss him, she reflected as she got into bed that night, she agreed that it sounded like the right choice for Michael.

September 1998

Frankie tried not to take the first tablet as soon as she got home from the pharmacy. But in the end, she only lasted a couple of hours.

And it helped.

Immediately.

But she knew that she needed to force herself to save the remaining ones for the flights.

And as she lay in bed that night, she thought about that thing Michael had asked her when he got back from his Easter retreat, in those awful weeks before the start of his A-Levels.

He'd come into her room as she was getting ready for bed. He'd been out all evening and she hadn't heard him come in.

'Hey,' she'd cried out in annoyance and elbowed him out of the way as she grabbed her dressing gown from the back of the door. 'Knock before you come barging in here.'

He'd ignored her and stared her straight in the eye.

'Why did you hate me?'

'What are you talking about? It's late. This is my room. Can we—'

'When I was a baby.'

And then he came right up to her and pushed her in the chest so that she stumbled into the bedside table.

'What kind of mother hates her baby?'

*

And then her brain started to slow down as if a cloud had passed over, rubbing out all the memories again, blurring his words with the features of his face as her breathing grew calm and she found herself falling into the deepest sleep she'd had in the best part of twenty years.

March 1997

Michael had agreed, reluctantly, to give his dad a hand getting the farm ready for the lambs during the Easter holidays. Just the odd day or two, here and there, to take a break from revision before the exams got under way. His father had been adamant that he'd pay Michael for his help – at least put a bit towards Michael's holiday fund; he knew how hard he'd been saving. It would be a chance to get a bit more driving practice under his belt too, and if the weather was good enough, he'd show him a good spot to catch barbel; they might even have time to go shooting. It would be fun.

'Basic life skills, really. I mean, it's all well and good being able to quote Corinthians, Mike, but it's not much use on an everyday basis. Trust me, girls like a man who knows what to do with his hands.'

Michael had grimaced. 'I'm not really into that sort of thing, Dad.'

'Nonsense, come on. I wouldn't be a proper dad, would I, if I didn't at least teach you *something* about the real world?'

Michael hadn't answered immediately. He didn't want to go; he hated the atmosphere on the farm and always slept badly there but he didn't know how to say any of that to his father. And so, instead, he agreed, and lied yet again to his mother, pretending he was going on an Easter retreat with the St Thomas's lot.

But he had the impression that she didn't believe him.

She was on her way out to work when he mentioned it, too casually, his back to her as he went upstairs.

'Hey, come back. We haven't finished speaking,' she'd said. 'What sort of retreat? Who else is going to be there?'

'I'll be back Monday.' He fiddled with the buttons on his watch. 'There's the vigil tomorrow that I'm helping with; we're walking down to Hinksey; Sami's going too. I think she's the only other one from school...' He trailed off.

'Okay,' his mother had said, a little uncertainly as she headed out the door. 'Leave the phone number for the place, though.'

His dad met him in town on the Thursday afternoon and Michael dutifully waited – his backpack crushed awkwardly against his shins under the table – for his father to drink two pints before he suggested they head back before it got dark. His dad didn't seem to want to speak much. He'd had the inspectors round, he explained as they went back to the car, and warned Michael that it was going to be a pretty heavy couple of days.

'But I just need to pop in on someone on the way,' he said, backing – too quickly – out of the parking bay. 'So we'll go via Cowley, if that's okay?'

'Who?' Michael asked.

'Oh, no-one you know. Shouldn't take long,' he added, as they headed out beyond the BMW plant, swerving down a no-through road lined with wild grass and flattened beer cans.

Michael's feet felt too cold. He stared out of the wing mirror to memorise the route, noting how all of the houses were identical, with their oppressive dark-brown brick fronts and matching window frames, which – with their gauzy white curtains – reminded Michael of a row of hooded eyes.

A Proper Mother

His father pulled up outside the house at the end of the road next to a skip filled with bags of builder's sand. On top, someone had dumped a dirty mattress and a toy pushchair with a wheel missing.

A woman opened the door. She was wearing thick blue eyeshadow, a purple velour tracksuit top and pristine Reebok trainers.

'Welcome, Mr Webb.' Her voice was solemn – unexpectedly deep.

Michael's father gestured to him. 'This is my son, Mike.' He whispered something in her ear, pressing a wad of cash into her hand.

'Welcome, Mr Webb,' she said again, to Michael this time, discreetly slipping the money into the back pocket of her jeans.

Michael nodded politely, noting the way that the woman's fringe, cut in a perfectly straight line, didn't move in time with her face – like a wig.

She led them into the house. It was hot inside and Michael was surprised at how lovely the music was that was playing – it sounded like glockenspiels and bells and it reminded him of that Javanese gamelan tape that Miss Albany had brought in for him. It seemed so out of place against the lilac floral wallpaper and thick synthetic carpet.

There was some sort of incense burning somewhere. It filled the air with a pungent vanilla scent that was too sweet and made Michael want to gag.

'You wait here a moment, Mike.' His father gestured to a small seating area at the bottom of the stairs. There were three red velvet-backed chairs in a row and a small glass side table with a pile of magazines on it.

Michael looked away. 'I might wait outside actually,' he said, turning back.

'No, you won't.' His father gripped his forearm. 'You'll wait here, like I said.' And then he smiled, his eyelids heavy from the beer, and went upstairs.

The woman reappeared with a tray.

But Michael shook his head and she went away.

Someone turned the music up so that it was much too loud. Michael stared straight ahead at a vase of plastic purple orchids, wishing more than anything that he was back home, having dinner with his mother.

When his father came down a few minutes later, he had lost the smile. 'Your turn now.'

'No thanks, Dad. I want to go home.'

'What's wrong with you?' his father hissed. 'A fricking fairy?'

'What?' Michael froze, his face reddening. He shook his head, trying to think of something to say back to his dad but all the words had dried up.

'I've already paid. Now get in there before I change my mind.' He pushed Michael towards the stairs.

The door was ajar. Michael hesitated in the doorway. The room was small, airless and dimly lit. It smelt of semen and sweat mixed up with that same vanilla stuff.

A woman was sitting on a red eiderdown on a narrow bed. She was wearing a short transparent black nightdress, lined with black furry pompoms along the hem, and black patent high-heels. There was a small stain the colour of dried blood on the carpet in front of her feet. The walls were bare. And in the corner of the room was an armchair with a black satin dressing gown draped over one arm.

'Hello,' she said blankly, watching him through a curtain of long black hair. She had thick white make-up on her face – and she was thin, like a child, so that the sinews and tendons of her wrists and ankles stood up from the flesh. The skin around her mouth was bumpy, sores still visible beneath layers of metallic plum lipstick. And above the shadow marking where her own eyebrows had once been she had painted fine reddish-brown semi-circles that made her look like a porcelain doll.

When she spoke again Michael realised she must have been older than he had initially thought – at least twenty-three or so.

'You're the same.' She gestured to her own cheekbones so that her hand covered her mouth. 'Like your dad.' She left her hand where it was and spoke loudly, to make herself heard over the music, her eyes devoid of all expression. 'He said you've never fucked nobody.'

Michael looked away. The muscles in his arms stiffened.

She looked just beyond him. 'You want to fuck, then? Deluxe, yeah?'

'No.' He shook his head emphatically and glanced behind him, wondering if anyone had overheard. He shut the door. His mouth felt dry and he pictured his father, leering at him. 'I don't want anything,' he snapped.

The woman shrugged, picking at a little scab on her knee. 'Okay. But it's the same price.' She sniffed. 'Deluxe, isn't it?' she said again, as she eyed him warily.

When Michael came out, it was raining. His father was gone and the woman was nowhere to be seen.

His dad didn't look at him when Michael climbed into the car, fists still clenched in his pockets, as if he were in possession of something special that he feared his father would take from him.

He started the engine before Michael had even had time to close the door.

'Like her, did you?'

Michael said nothing.

'I warned her you wouldn't know an arse from an elbow.'

His neck hurt on one side.

'You're a prig, aren't you? Like your mum.' His father stared straight ahead, fiddling with the radio until he landed on Classic FM.

And then he drove back to the farm, the only conversation the whimsical soliloquies of the radio host above the squeaking of the windscreen wipers, every time there was a lull in the music.

Although Michael thanked him for driving, when he eventually spotted a sign to Misselden, his father didn't reply, swerving wide down the middle of the quiet country lanes to blunt the corners, as if he couldn't wait for the journey to be over.

As they pulled up at the farm, a piano started playing – so gently that it was as if it were playing for them alone. Michael recognised it immediately; it was Entr'acte from *Carmen*; they'd played it in orchestra and the opening always disoriented him, no matter how many times he heard it.

Neither of them got out.

Instead, without saying anything, his father turned the volume up and they stared, straight ahead, at the old barn.

And as the flute climbed higher Michael heard him sniff, catching out of the corner of his eye the movement of his father's sleeve.

But he held his breath and didn't dare look over at him.

After they'd eaten, Michael's father came back to the table with a bottle of whisky and offered it to Michael.

Michael shook his head. He glanced at the clock. It was only half-past eight. It would be a good two hours before he'd be able to escape to bed.

'So tomorrow, you're okay to get cracking on the fences, like we said? In the side barn, you know, where Ray keeps the JCBs. That way I can finish off the isolation stuff with the inspectors.'

'Okay.'

'You alright, Mike?'

'Yes,' he said coldly, looking away.

'It's a great help, Mike. Couldn't do it without you – not this weekend. Hope I haven't dragged you away from anything more exciting?'

'Not really,' he said warily.

'Not got a girlfriend or anything, Mike?' His father poured himself a glass.

Michael flushed and shook his head.

'How about your mum? Up to anything nice this weekend?'

'I'm not sure actually.'

'She seeing anyone at the moment? She still fooling around with that Carmichael guy from the surgery?'

Michael shrugged and looked away.

'Does she ever talk about me?' He was watching Michael's reaction so carefully that he accidentally missed the edge of the glass. 'You know – why she left; that sort of stuff?'

Michael got up to fetch a cloth. 'Yes, sometimes,' he lied, studiously keeping his eyes fixed on the table as he wiped up the sticky mess.

'Oh?' His father sat very still.

'She said you sort of went your separate ways,' Michael ventured, retreating into the kitchen.

'Did she?' He snorted. 'That's one way of putting it, I suppose.'

When Michael came back his father was staring down at his glass, deep in thought.

He noticed that the piano was closed and there was a box of sheet music resting on the stool. 'Do you mind if I...?'

'Go ahead. Just shove all that stuff on the floor. It needs tuning, mind, but the guy's booked up until June.' He sat back and yawned.

Michael started to play with one hand, absent-mindedly leafing through a pile of sheet music with the other until he found that old black and white edition of Schumann's *Kinderszenen*. Halfway through he paused and lifted the lid of the piano to release one of the hammers that had got stuck.

His father was silent.

When he finished playing his dad still didn't say anything. Michael stood up, pretending to look for something else to play. His ears felt hot.

He glanced over his shoulder. His dad was staring down at his hands, so still that Michael wondered if he had fallen asleep.

'You alright, Dad?'

'What? Oh yeah, I was just thinking about that thing we were talking about. That was lovely, by the way. I used to play that when I was your age.'

'Oh, right.' Michael felt the corners of his mouth pulling downwards.

'I can't blame her, really. Everyone warned me she wouldn't last five minutes on a farm. But you know better, don't you? When you're young.'

Michael stared at the elaborate Gothic German script on the cover as he tried to distract himself from what his father was saying.

'She shouldn't have strung it out as long as she did.' He sighed loudly. 'But she's a bit of a wuss, your mum, isn't she?'

'I think she was just trying to do her best,' Michael whispered, hardly daring to move.

'Is that so?'

It felt like hours before his dad spoke again.

'Well, perhaps I didn't handle her as well as I could have done. But she was all over the place when she was expecting. And it's no secret that you came as a bit of a... how shall we put it...?'

Eventually Michael turned to look at him.

'A surprise.' His dad was watching him, a darkness in his eyes that Michael hadn't seen before, as if they didn't reflect the light properly, but swallowed it all up instead. 'Not mistake, as such.'

Michael's stomach churned. Out of the corner of his eye he saw the gun cabinet and pictured it swinging open on its hinges.

'But she didn't want it. Sorry – not *it* – you, rather.' He gave a strange smile, as if he were taking pleasure in watching his son grow upset. 'Still wanted the other one.'

Michael sat down heavily so that the piano stool creaked. He clung to the underside of the stool, trying to flex his fingers. He felt a sense of dread stirring inside him. 'What are you talking about?'

'It doesn't matter. Wasn't meant to be. But it upset her. Upset both of us, if I'm honest. She lost her spark. Even when you came along so soon afterwards.'

Michael concentrated on following the curling tail of the treble clef with his eyes. But from nowhere he saw that woman again – the expression on her face and the way she had looked at him as he left the room. He needed to get out of there.

'Do you know what she did? When you were a couple of days old, Mike? To think... if that guy hadn't got there when he did... There's no knowing what would have happened.'

Michael tried to stand but his legs buckled. He grabbed hold of the piano for balance, clutching the keys in a loud discordant panic as he turned to stagger towards the door.

'She tried to kill you, Mike.'

Michael felt a loud ringing in his ears. He saw his father get up and although his mouth was moving Michael couldn't hear anything he was saying.

It was as if there were a screen between them, and as his father reached out to put an arm around him, he reminded Michael of a mime artist, pressing his hands against the glass.

Michael lay in the spare bed, thinking about what his father had said. Above the hammering rain he could hear something in the yard. He listened. It didn't sound altogether human. And then he heard a baby crying.

He opened the window and the rain blew in, soaking the hems of the thin white nylon curtains and gathering, in a narrow pool, on the windowsill, in which – on its back – a dead bluebottle floated. Michael shivered. It must have been cats fighting.

It was so dark – the moon buried in cloud, as if it had been abandoned there. He leant right out to listen – water running down the back of his neck until he was quite sure there was nothing there.

He got back into bed.

But as he fell asleep, he was certain he heard it again, in the back of his mind, getting closer now. And he woke, abruptly, to find his body lurching downwards, paralysed by that shallow ferocious sleep that he had known since childhood. And sensing, instantly, that very strong presence: there was someone in the room with him.

And then he saw it – a figure – emerging, rustling – from the darkness.

He tried to scream but his jaw was locked.

It was a woman – her face absent – almost entirely concealed in a vast black hood – with only the eyes visible, from the glint of her tears.

He scrunched his eyes tightly shut and tried to shout out but his face was stuck, rigid, and his throat felt all tied up – so that the only sound it allowed out was a strangled reedy whine.

She came closer, with that same soft crackling sound, like cellophane.

He could feel her standing right next to him, leaning over his body. Something cool brushed his face.

He couldn't open his eyes. His whole body was shaking. And he couldn't tell whether it was the dream or the woman that was causing him to rock like that, from side to side, so that his shoulder and his jaw were pressed, at once, into the bedding.

And then he heard something snap.

His body loosened and he started to come to. He opened his eyes and the darkness immediately dispersed as he realised that the landing light was on.

The next day Michael got up early, remembering, abstractly, that it was Good Friday. His father had already gone and Michael was taken aback to see that the door to the gun cabinet was ajar.

He edged towards it and took the case out, turning it over very delicately in his hand, glancing over his shoulder to check there was no-one there. His heart was beating too fast and although he knew it was silly to be afraid – the gun probably wasn't even assembled – he still handled the case very carefully, as if it might have contained a grenade.

The gun wasn't loaded. He took the pieces out and laid them on the kitchen table. The barrel was much shorter than on the one his father had shown him. But the safety mechanism was identical. He checked it – twice – like his father had demonstrated, before closing the empty case and putting it back in the cabinet.

He wasn't sure what to do with the pieces but he knew it wasn't safe to leave them there. So he carried them up to the spare room, wrapped them carefully in his pyjamas and put them in his backpack, positioning them securely between his history textbook and his clarinet case. He'd get rid of them somehow.

Before leaving he scribbled a little note for his father and left it on the kitchen table, propped against a box of Shredded Wheat. *Thanks for having me to stay, Dad. I'm not feeling well today so I thought I'd head off early and get some rest. Sorry to leave you in the lurch.*

He bit his lip.

And then he started to head home.

He knew the buses would be all over the place with it being the bank holiday weekend but the Liturgy wasn't until midday so he had plenty of time. Besides, he wasn't sure if he felt like going or whether he'd even feel welcome there anymore, let alone be able to concentrate on the service. So he walked and walked, and after a couple of hours, when he was tired and thirsty and ready to give up, he got on the first available bus back to town.

He went down to the canal and sat on a rotting wooden bench by the rubbish bins to watch the dragonflies hover and skim over the scummy surface of the water. He often sat in that spot in the early evening, watching the water change by the tiniest gradations of colour, as the sun fell away, its daily sacrifice, before humbly rising again.

He looked down at the rubbish caught in the weeds – cans and sweet wrappers and a tube of grey concertinaed plastic that looked like it had been ripped off a tumble drier – thinking deeply about those things his father had said.

It was too much to make sense of – all at once – and he was worried that he wasn't going to be able to cope with it all.

But it seemed to resolve something that he had always suspected rather than known – that something so pure could never come from something so foul.

He checked his watch. It was ten past three; the service would be over.

He opened his backpack, patting the clothing to check the pieces of the gun underneath. He felt suddenly queasy and his heart was racing.

He took out his clarinet case and looked all around him.

The canal path was empty.

The velvet was worn thin. He stayed there a while, the midges gathering just above his head. And then he took the pieces of the clarinet out of the case, one by one, and before he had time to really question himself any further on the matter, he hurled them into the water.

September 1998

Frankie took the next tablet the minute she reached the airport, at half-past four in the morning, not anticipating for a moment that the flight would be so extraordinarily delayed. She curled up in a corner seat in the departure lounge with a copy of the airline magazine that had been left on the seat beside her, resting her head on Olivia's turquoise travel pillow.

She stared at the woman on the cover.

It struck her that she had been so fixated on the journey that she hadn't really given much attention to the thought that in a matter of hours she would be there – in that strange place with the sort of sea that you only ever see on holiday programmes on the TV.

The woman's hair was still dry and her teeth gleamed as she patiently taught someone else's child to swim alongside her.

Frankie tossed the magazine aside and closed her eyes, letting her mind wander, trying not to think back to that dreadful time before Michael's exams as she felt herself physically tumbling, first into a dull, medicated sleep, before falling headlong into a black, dreamless hole.

April 1997

Although Frankie knew that Michael just wanted to do his best, she nevertheless thought his study regime was excessive. After all, hadn't everyone known, practically since he was born, that he would excel at everything he ever tried? It hardly seemed necessary to spend all of that time revising.

'But I've been given so much,' he explained, craned over his Bible and his Greek and history textbooks. 'It wouldn't be right not to give everything back.'

And so, on the first day of term, when he didn't come down for breakfast, she was worried that he'd finally made himself ill. She went upstairs to check on him, pushing gently, when he didn't answer, against his bedroom door.

The room was empty.

She looked around. The bed was made. His books were on the floor and the window was closed. She cast her mind back to the previous day. He'd been rather subdued – ever since he got back from his Easter retreat, come to think of it – but she had assumed he was just nervous about the impending exams and hadn't thought much more of it. And then he'd got changed and gone out, almost immediately, to help Monira at the homeless shelter, saying that he wanted to take his mind off everything so he could wake up fresh the next morning. She realised she hadn't seen him after that. She'd gone to bed early, and had just assumed he must have come in after she'd gone up. She felt her breathing quicken. Had he not been back at all?

And then she spotted a piece of paper, folded in half, on the pillow.

It was addressed to Frances.

She opened it – her hands trembling so hard that she could barely read the lines of tiny disordered handwriting. She sat down heavily on the bed, her stomach dropping, and pins and needles coursing ferociously down one of her arms.

I'm going away for a while. I need to be alone. I don't think I can be who everyone else needs me to be.

Beneath, he had copied out a verse from the Bible in tiny letters with quotation marks.

'Though I have the gift of prophecy, and understand all mysteries, and all knowledge; and though I have all faith, so that I could remove mountains, and have not charity, I am nothing.'

She turned it around, and read it again, and a third time, but it still made no sense.

She grabbed her shoes and ran out into the road. She had forgotten to fasten one of them properly and slipped, falling hard on one arm. A car braked loudly and hooted but she didn't even see it.

'Michael!' She stumbled, trying to get up – dimly aware that she wasn't embarrassed, for once.

'Michael!' she hollered.

But he wasn't there.

She ran back inside and phoned John. He answered with a croak. 'Mum, it's seven o'clock—'

She heard someone in the background.

'Is that Michael with you?' she blurted.

'No, Mum.' He laughed awkwardly. 'It's... um... it's Liv.' He whispered something to someone.

'Olivia?' She momentarily forgot all about Michael. 'Oh, right. Sorry... I...' She changed gear. 'It doesn't matter. Have you seen Michael?'

'No.' He was alert now. 'Where is he?'

'I don't know.' She was breathing too fast. 'He's done something stupid. I know he has. John, you've got to—'

'Mum,' he said slowly. 'Calm down. Everything's okay. I'm coming round.'

She heard what sounded like a whine of protest from Olivia but John ignored her.

'John,' Frankie wailed. 'What if he...' But she couldn't think it, let alone say it.

'Try to relax. Have a cup of tea. I'll be there in a couple of hours.'

'No.' She stood up. 'That's too long. I can't wait here. I've got to find him. What if he needs me?'

She knew it was probably pointless but she flicked through the phone book to find the number for Monira at the homeless shelter. There was no reply but she scribbled the number down on a scrap of paper and shoved it in her wallet, grabbing her keys and getting straight in the car.

But she had barely started the ignition when she saw it.

A white Land Rover.

It was parked at the end of the street and the driver's door opened. She could only see his leg as he planted one boot on the road but she knew it was Callum.

She immediately locked her door and tried to steady her breathing.

But he didn't look up at her. Instead, he went around to the passenger seat and Frankie saw there was someone else in the car. She sat back in her seat and gave a deep sigh.

It was Michael.

He wasn't dead.

And she closed her eyes – allowing herself, for a moment, to forget even that her husband was actually there, right in front of her, after all those years of imagining it – so immense was her relief that her son was still alive.

Callum helped Michael climb out of the car. He appeared to be wrapped in some sort of duvet or quilt with no cover on. It was yellow and stained and Michael's hair was wet, slicked flat against his head.

Michael looked at the ground as he hobbled towards her, leaning against Callum who – a look of solemn concentration on his face – supported their son with one arm around his waist, never once taking his eyes off Frankie.

Callum looked slim and very tanned and she instinctively checked her appearance in the rear-view mirror as she got out of the car. Her hand was shaking as she locked the car door.

'Michael,' she called out, her voice wavering. 'Where have you been?'

'Hello, Frances.' Callum lay a hand on her waist. 'God, you look awful. You must have been worried sick.'

She flushed.

'And what's this?' He reached for her hand before she could tell what he was doing and lifted it gently. His hands were warm. 'Have you hurt—?'

She snatched her hand away, glancing down at her grazed forearm. It was bleeding.

'Where was he?'

'Wait,' he mouthed. 'Let's get him warm and dry first.' He walked past her towards the house.

Michael walked as if asleep. He didn't seem aware that she was even there. Or if he was, he didn't acknowledge her.

Callum gestured to her to hand him the house keys and she hesitated before obeying.

*

Callum looked around, eyebrows raised. He bent down to pick up an electoral campaign leaflet from the doormat.

She ignored him. 'Michael, do you want to go and have a lie down?'

Michael didn't respond. Instead, he stood, hunched in the hallway, staring at the carpet. He was leaning slightly to one side and at one point he swayed towards the wall so that she had to reach out to grab him under the arms to prevent him from toppling over.

His tee-shirt was damp and his skin smelt so sour she had to turn her face as she edged him towards the stairs, looking back nervously over her shoulder as Callum picked up a little photo frame on the side table. It was a picture Bobbi had sent her – of Frankie with John and Michael and Bobbi's girls – at the beach at Aberporth when the children were tiny; it was so cold that the waterfall had frozen over.

Michael was so unresponsive it seemed to take forever to get him up the stairs.

She could hear Callum in the kitchen now. And then she heard him unlock the back door.

'Come on, Michael,' she said, her ears hot. It felt like hauling a bag of cement. And when she finally helped him to collapse on the bed, she realised she was sweating.

He turned on one side and closed his eyes.

She waited for a moment and crouched down beside him. She laid a hand softly on his cheek. He was very cold. And it seemed, from the quiet of his breathing, as though he had fallen straight to sleep. She tucked the duvet around him and covered him in a blanket, as if she were trying to conceal something.

And then she knelt, very still, beside the bed, with her eyes closed, where she stayed for as long as she could before eventually going back downstairs to face her husband.

Callum was sitting at the kitchen table, doing the crossword. He'd made himself a cup of coffee. In front of him, in the middle of the table, stood a huge bouquet of fresh roses, lilies and chrysanthemums in a tall Art Deco vase that had been a wedding present from Bobbi and Al. To one side, encrusted in dark green sludge, lay the large pair of pinking shears from the sewing box in the living room.

Confused, she looked out of the window at the raised beds in the far corner of the garden.

He'd cut down all her flowers.

She snatched the scissors, gripping the blades in her fist.

'What are you doing here?' Her voice was low and unsteady.

He took a sip and wrote something down neatly in the grid, a pleased smile on his face. 'Oatmeal,' he said.

'What did you do to him?'

'Hey.' He raised his hands in mock surrender. She noticed that he obviously hadn't shaved for a couple of days, observing, in spite of herself, how much it suited him and almost not spotting the little cut that ran along his jawbone. His dark hair was flecked with grey at the sides now, too, she realised. But the eyes were unchanged. They rolled, unseeing, all over her – up and down – almost as if they could reach right inside her.

She crossed her arms and sat down opposite him, feeling the heat rising up her throat.

'I hadn't heard a peep from him since last week. He was giving me a hand on Thursday and said he'd stick around a couple of days but he vanished first thing next morning. Left me in the shit, to be perfectly honest with you. I tried to get hold of him but no luck. Next I know – middle of the night – some woman on the phone from Thames Valley Police. Says they'd found some lad in Florence Park acting weird; some dog walker something or other; thought he was a druggie. Anyway, took him into the station last night – pretty incoherent by all accounts – and then he mentions Andy. Remember Andy Caulfield?'

Frankie stared at him, baffled. 'Andy Caulfield? What on earth has *he* got to do with it?'

'I don't know. Anyway, he called me, obviously, so I drove over first thing.'

'What was he doing in the park? Had he been at church? Did he go there after the retreat?'

'What retreat? Oh, who knows what he was thinking. He wasn't talking much.' He frowned and looked her up and down. 'God, look at you. I thought *I* was tired.'

She tucked her hair behind her ear instinctively, hating herself in the same moment for doing so. She swallowed. She could taste the acid in the back of her throat.

He looked down at the paper. 'Five across in eight,' he mumbled. 'Four blanks c. Potion confused dim niece.' He paused. 'Anagram of dim niece – must be.'

She stared at him. 'Medicine,' she said.

He smiled, picking up the pencil. 'Haven't lost your touch, then.'

She pictured that awful night back at the farm; it was a few days after Christmas, shortly before she'd left Callum for good. Michael was not yet one. She'd called the police. When she heard a car pull up outside, she'd crept downstairs in her nightie, still carrying Michael – John clinging to her in silence. She waited in the hallway, listening at the door, alarmed to hear voices and loud laughter.

And then someone put a record on – it was the Doors – the needle falling clumsily in the middle of 'Alabama Song' so that she heard it bounce, far too loud, already. She peered through the crack in the door – pressing her hand, too hard, against the back of Michael's head to protect him – bewildered to see Andy, John's old school friend, at the record player, in his police uniform, sifting through Callum's LPs while Callum fetched him a beer.

'How does Michael know that man?' she asked now.

He shrugged but didn't look up.

She pictured herself jumping on him and pushing the blades clean through his neck but as he sat, his face in his hands, concentrating on the clues in front of him, all she could see was Michael.

Callum gave a big yawn, and when he spoke again, he looked suddenly very sad. 'He was saying all sorts of rubbish, they said – something about a dragon. The woman asked me if he was schizophrenic.'

'What?' She peered at him, incredulous, through her tears. The room seemed to grow darker. 'Why would he say all that?'

'I don't know. Maybe because there's something true there, deep down. I told him how much you hated...' he paused, staring right through her, '... *me*, mainly. But him even more.'

'No.' She shook her head vehemently.

'I should never have said it. About that time you tried to—'

'No!' She was shaking all over now. 'How dare you? Why did...' But the words wouldn't come out properly and she knew she had to get out of the room.

'You know I hate secrets. They tear families apart.'

'We're not a family!' she screamed. 'Why won't you leave us alone? How could you...?' Her shoulders were heaving and her hands were wet. She looked down to see a fine red cut that ran along her palm, as if to stop her lifeline short. She clamped her fingers down to the heel of her hand to stop the flow. 'Get out,' she growled.

He pretended he hadn't heard her. 'He was upset—'

'Get out!' she yelled, pointing the blades directly at his face.

'Okay, relax, I'm going.' He reached across and ripped the cover page off the newspaper, folding it roughly and scoring a line with the end of the pencil, leaving a thick yellow line across Tony Blair's smile. Then he tore the crossword out, folded it, and put it in the breast pocket of his shirt.

'I'm sorry.' He stood up straight.

She looked away but he caught her, from behind, in an unexpected embrace.

'I really am, you know.'

She froze but he held his face there – warm – against hers so that she couldn't help but breathe in a scent of something familiar – like ginger laced with lime.

'God, I miss you sometimes,' he whispered, his breath hot in her ear.

And she almost let herself lean back into him, just for a moment, before she snapped to her senses and pulled away.

'I'm sorry.' He sat back down. 'Don't know why I did that. I'm a bit all over the place to tell the truth.'

She waited.

'We've had a… I don't know how to say it… a situation… on the farm.'

'What do you mean a situation?'

'Ray found one of the cows. Last week.' He sliced the air across his throat with his finger. 'They think she was infected.'

She stared at him.

'You don't mean—'

He nodded, his mouth downturned. He twisted his hands together.

'How do you know that's what it was?'

'We don't. Don't know anything yet. She's been taken away for testing. We'll find out next couple of days, I'd have thought. But I've got a bad feeling about it.'

'Why?'

He squinted. 'A few things weren't right, looking back. It's only when you put them together it starts to make sense, isn't it? Her milk was down. Ray mentioned it – couple of times. I should have twigged. And then she was sick one morning. Very. Thought it was something got into the feed but I should have given it more thought.' He shook his head. 'Nothing else to speak of, though. Maybe it's nothing…'

She looked away. 'And if it does turn out to be that?' she ventured.

He stared at her as if the enormity of it all were only just starting to dawn on him. 'Well, it's curtains, isn't it?'

Neither of them said anything.

And when Callum spoke again, his voice was too small, as if it belonged to someone else. 'You've got to square up to this stuff, though, haven't you? Even if it's hard.' He looked at her, as if he wasn't sure he believed it anymore.

She nodded doubtfully.

He pushed the chair back. 'Okay, I'm off now.'

She tried to say something but a sudden memory derailed her of one morning, years before, when she'd been pregnant with Michael. She'd come looking for him in the main barn, John beside her, holding her hand. They'd seen Lulu the sheepdog lying on the floor of the barn, waiting for him to say goodbye to the lambs who were off to slaughter. Lulu had leapt up excitedly when she saw John but Callum had been so embarrassed when he turned to find them there. 'Christ, what's wrong with me?' He had laughed, coming over and crouching down to kiss John on the top of his head. 'All this fuss over some bloody sheep. I'm worse than you, mate.'

She hesitated before reaching out to embrace him. 'Good luck.' She squeezed his shoulders. 'Let me know if...' she trailed off.

'If what?' He pulled away. 'If I need a hand incinerating any livestock?' He laughed. 'No offence, but you'd be quite far down my list of people to call on.'

She folded her arms, feeling all the blood rush to her face. 'Oh, just go, why don't you.'

She slammed the door behind him and waited in the hallway until her breathing had returned to normal. She didn't move until she was absolutely certain that the car she had heard driving away was his.

September 1998

When the announcement eventually came – over eleven hours after she had arrived at the airport – that the aircraft was preparing to land, Frankie thought she was going to implode from a toxic combination of anxiety and relief. She rested her forehead, eyes closed, against the clammy seat in front, clinging so tightly with both hands that she accidentally pulled the hair of the woman in front, who cried out in surprise – the same woman who had had to wake her up in the airport lounge, Frankie realised in dismay, shrinking down in her seat, even more mortified than before.

As she stepped out of the air-conditioned aeroplane she was struck immediately by a wall of dusky blue heat. She gasped. Even though it was almost six o'clock in the evening it was still like standing under a hairdrier. She looked across the concourse. The airport building sat in a wobbling sea of concrete and tarmac behind a row of red and blue Aegean Airlines planes.

Inside the terminal the air was cool but prickly and she could almost smell the heat trying to force its way in. She felt a thrill of excitement as she walked down a corridor past a room – glassed off – packed full of people waiting.

She dutifully stood in line to show her passport, wondering briefly if Michael had passed that way on his travels, imagining what he'd say if he were there alongside her now.

It was eight o'clock by the time the minibus dropped Frankie at her taverna – Delfini Studios, it was called – a small blue and white painted block with individual balconies – and covered, all down one side, in a cascade of dark pink bougainvillea.

A woman – in her seventies or thereabouts – came out to meet Frankie off the bus. She had short dark hair and was wearing a black and white sleeveless floral dress and white pumps. She was holding a handwritten sign with Frankie's name on it and she greeted Frankie enthusiastically in Greek, introducing herself as Maria and clutching her so hard by the upper arms when she embraced her that her fingertips left a mark. Her nose was crooked and she had high cheekbones with eyes that were bright and rounded under the lids.

And Frankie followed her.

April 1997

After Callum had left, Frankie had gone up to check on Michael.

He was still asleep.

So she went back downstairs and was surprised to find John standing in the hallway.

'Oh, John, I meant to call you.'

His hair had grown and was streaked with blond from the sun. He looked suspiciously clean, in his oversized bright blue Zuma Jay surfing tee-shirt and baggy jeans, and furious under his deep tan.

'Thank you for coming.' She sat down on the stairs, suddenly overwhelmed with exhaustion.

He smelt strongly of that Hugo Boss aftershave – the specific one that his friend Dominic had apparently got for his birthday and which John had spent hours trying to locate – occupying most of the staff of the Croydon branch of Boots, by all accounts, as they hunted for the last bottle from the depths of the stock room – while Frankie waited outside in the boiling-hot car on the way home from IKEA.

'Thanks,' he said tersely. 'I take it you found Michael then. I passed Dad on the way. That was a nice surprise.'

'I'm sorry, John,' she said wearily.

'Sometimes I think you're all on another fucking planet.' He stormed into the kitchen. 'Wouldn't it cross your mind, just once, to think about how I might feel?'

Through the doorway she watched him go straight to the fridge.

'I've just driven like a maniac to get here. We were supposed to go to Liv's parents for the weekend. We had loads of stuff planned so they're all *really* pissed off with me – understandably. And then I get here and – surprise, surprise – he's here all along, but no-one bothered to mention it. Well, you know what?' He grabbed the orange juice and lifted it to his lips. 'You can all fuck off,' he said through a mouth full of juice.

Frankie didn't say anything.

She just waited, watching a trickle of juice run down John's neck, for him to finish drinking.

The entire carton.

Straight from the carton.

She still didn't say anything when he slammed it back in the fridge and leant against the sink, his back to her, looking out of the window.

'Is he okay?' he said, in a very small voice.

She hauled herself up, retrieved the empty carton from the fridge and threw it in the bin. She put her arm around his shoulder. 'He's had a really bad night. I'm not sure what happened exactly. He's having a sleep.'

John sniffed. 'I was so worried… when you called.' He let out a huge sob. 'I thought I was going to crash the car.'

She hugged him hard.

'I thought he'd—'

'Don't, John.' She squeezed her eyes shut.

He wiped his face with his sleeve. 'I thought, what if I can't get there in time? And then when I saw Dad's car…'

She felt him shudder.

'It's okay, John.'

He pulled away. 'That fucking idiot. I can't believe he'd do something so stupid. Does that kid ever think about anyone except himself?'

'Hey, calm down.' She drew him back in and held him until he was still. 'Why don't you go up? He's pretty washed out – just to warn you. Go easy on him.'

He hesitated and she caught the look of fear in his eyes.

She squeezed his hand. 'Let's go together.'

She waited in the doorway while John sat down on the bed.

'It's just me,' he said, his voice wobbling. He cleared his throat, reached out and lay a hand on his brother's shoulder.

Michael let out a strange moan, like an injured animal.

'You had us scared there, mate.' John's voice broke. 'Don't do that shit again.' He bit his lip. 'You could come and stay with me for a couple of days, if things are tough here.'

Michael made no sound as John sat motionless.

It was so quiet that Frankie thought Michael must have fallen asleep again, but just as she turned away to go back downstairs there was a rustling, as he started to sit up, very stiffly, as if all his limbs ached. His eyes were open just a crack and he looked right at her as if he didn't recognise her before very slowly reaching out and folding his thin arms around John's shoulders, allowing his head to fall, heavy, on his brother's chest, like a sleeping child.

When Michael finally emerged from his room, not long after John had left, he had such dark shadows under his eyes that he looked as though he had aged ten years.

He didn't speak for a couple of hours. And then, just before going back up to bed, he stared into Frankie's eyes as if he were searching for something.

He turned away.

'They were burning all the cows,' he said, his voice deeper than normal, growly. 'A few fields along from Dad's.'

'Oh, Michael.' She tried to hug him but he shrugged her off.

'The smell.' He turned away; his chest heaved involuntarily. 'All the way down the lane. Some of them were still alive – must have known what was coming – that smell – couldn't have been anything else. Like burning rubber; chemicals or something; but this weird sweetness at the same time.'

He stopped and stared at her again.

She felt her face tremble. 'I'm so sorry you saw all that.'

He looked down at his hands and when he spoke again his voice came out in a whisper. 'Why didn't you tell me all that stuff? Why I didn't belong; where I came from?'

'What do you mean?' She stepped backwards.

'You always kept me from Dad. Made me afraid of him.' He looked her bravely in the eye. 'You don't tell the truth, do you?' His voice hardened. 'What did I ever do to you? Why did you hate me?'

'I didn't hate you, Michael,' she sobbed. 'I didn't keep anything from—'

'I'm sorry if I ruined everything for you.'

'Oh, Michael. You haven't ruined anything. What are you talking about?'

He looked away. 'I heard you, Frances. Saw you crying. But I didn't understand.'

She grabbed him by the arms. 'What are you talking about, Michael?'

He pulled away.

'I love you, Michael. I want to help; I wish I understood what was wrong.'

His eyes narrowed. 'You don't love me,' he said.

She stepped back.

'I don't think you've ever loved me.'

She gripped him by the arm, the tears falling more freely now, so that her shoulders heaved.

But he wrenched himself free.

'Don't say those things, Michael,' she hissed, bowing her head to hide her face.

'It's okay to tell the truth, Frances, even if people don't like it.'

'But it's not the truth,' she snapped.

His mouth was twisted. 'It's good to hate, sometimes, isn't it?'

She shook him by the shoulders.

'No.' He pushed her, hard, in the chest. 'Leave me alone.'

She gasped. 'What's wrong, Michael? Why are you talking like this?'

But he gazed at the air just above her as if he were watching something that only he could see.

The next day, he was up early and when he came upstairs to say goodbye, she was still in her dressing gown and overcome with relief that he was still there and looking so peaceful. The colour had almost fully returned to his face.

But when he spoke, it was with that same formality of the day before.

As if a light had gone out, behind the eyes.

'Don't suppose I could borrow the spare keys, could I? Can't find mine anywhere.'

'Of course.' She swallowed hard and made herself smile. 'They're just on the side table. Now go on.' She hugged him awkwardly. 'This is a big term for you. Go do your stuff.'

And although she tried once or twice in the weeks that followed, she couldn't find the right words, after that, to mention any of it again.

So, she didn't.

And nor did Michael.

Instead, they just carried on as if nothing had happened.

And before they knew it, the exams had come and gone and Michael was free at last to focus on his travels.

With the exception of a rather cryptic letter – a rambling rhapsody on the pitfalls of the monastic life, peppered with extensive quotations from Corinthians, weighing up the virtues of a daily discipline of cloistered prayer set against one of practical, community-based charity – and a single incoherent phone call, late one night, with the charges reversed, Frankie heard almost nothing from Michael in the weeks that followed his exams.

He had said in passing, shortly before he left home, that he thought he might travel for several months. But he had never provided further detail. And he was so decidedly evasive in his every communication, in fact, especially when it came to the subject of John and Olivia's engagement, that she sometimes wondered whether he even received her letters, let alone read any of them.

Despite Frankie's concerns that they were far too young to settle down, John and Olivia were adamant that they wanted to get married, agreeing eventually to a long engagement to really think about things first and give themselves plenty of time to get the details just right. They had set a very provisional date for the following December – Olivia having apparently always dreamt of a winter wedding and with firm opinions on John's shortlist of candidates for best man. Surely he agreed that it was better if it were someone who knew them both equally?

On Frankie's insistence, John finally agreed to write to Michael, too, to let him know that although he'd obviously like his brother to be his best man, he and Olivia would understand entirely if Michael wasn't comfortable with the idea. But that they'd appreciate it if he could let them know as soon as possible. He wrote to Michael twice, in fact – trying him at both the youth hostel in Sarria and the monastery on Kalymnos, just to be on the safe side.

But there was no response.

Frankie had mentioned it, too, in one of her first letters as soon as they'd got engaged back in July, a couple of weeks after Michael had left home, knowing how difficult it would be to contact him once he reached Egypt. She was sure he'd write to John.

Still, she reasoned, there was no law saying he had to congratulate his brother or anything. And what more could she do about it? After all, it wasn't really her responsibility, when all was said and done.

It was the not knowing that was so infuriating. It reminded her of the days leading up to her own wedding, marred by the foolish hope that her mum would turn up after all. In the end her mum had sent a card wishing her the best of luck for her special day, explaining that although she'd wanted to be there, of course, she hadn't wanted to get in the way, knowing how busy Frankie was bound to be. Hadn't wanted to cause any upset.

Frankie had torn it up before she'd even finished reading it.

But it had ruined everything.

She'd had to reapply all her make-up, arriving at the church almost fifteen minutes late in the end, so worried that people would be able to see that her eyes were still red.

It was John she felt sorry for, though. Because although John never mentioned Michael in company – especially not in front of Brian and Susanna – unless to refer to his brother's travels, or 'the gap year from hell', as he and Olivia called it – he complained to Frankie in private that he thought his brother's behaviour was out of order. And although Frankie knew he agreed with her that the main thing was that Michael was safe and that although it obviously wouldn't be up everyone's street at least Michael seemed – from what they could gather, amidst his rapturous reveries of pilgrimages and mountaintop retreats – to be having a nice time, he'd hurt John's feelings. She could tell.

So, it came as quite a surprise when late one evening in the middle of September there was a knock at the door. Frankie was ten minutes from the end of a particularly nerve-wracking episode of *Inspector Morse* and when she got up to see who it was, she was horrified to see a police car outside.

September 1998

Maria, the landlady, showed Frankie to her room – on the ground floor, as Frankie had specifically and repeatedly requested when she'd booked it – a large whitewashed room with a double mattress on the floor and an adjacent shower room that was miniature and spotless. And when the woman opened the sliding doors on to the hot stillness of the evening, against the deafening chorus of cicadas, gesturing proudly to the little courtyard area outside, especially reserved for Frankie, full of flowers, with a table and two chairs and a blue and white checked tablecloth, Frankie felt something lift from her body – like a physical release as her shoulders dropped and her legs seemed to strengthen beneath her.

She breathed in deeply, the evening giving way to an overpowering wild aroma, amplified by the darkness – a fusion of oregano, pine, sage and oranges – that took her straight back to her honeymoon. It was as if someone had reached down from a great height and carefully eased off all those years of tension that she had been carrying ever since, and rolled them into the sea.

September 1997

Frankie could clearly see the outline of two people through the glass – a man and a woman – both apparently in uniform. She opened the door.

The woman was tall – in her late twenties, probably – with dark hair and freckles, while her colleague was older – mid-fifties – with skin the colour of church candles and teeth to match.

'Good evening.' The male officer extended his hand while the woman held back, watching Frankie's reaction. 'Mrs Webb, is it? Sorry to disturb you this time of night. But we were wondering if we could have a few words with your son, Mike?'

'Do you mean Michael? He's not here. Why do you want to see him?'

'Would you mind telling us where we might find him, Mrs Webb?'

'He's away – abroad.'

'Are you saying he's fled the country, Mrs Webb?' He exchanged a glance with his colleague.

'No, of course not.' Frankie laughed. 'Not like that. I mean he's travelling. Well, on holiday. An Interrailing type thing...' She trailed off.

The female officer raised one eyebrow. 'Where is he now, Mrs Webb?'

'I'm not entirely sure,' she stuttered. 'Greece, I think.'

'You *think* you know what country your teenage son is in?' she said, in a loud voice. 'Have we got that right?'

Frankie bristled. 'Yes, he's travelling around. I've got a postcard somewhere from a few weeks ago. I don't think he mentioned where he was going next, though, or particular dates or anything.'

They were staring very solemnly at her as if they didn't believe her. The woman looked up as if to check the upstairs window locks. 'Can we come in, Mrs Webb?'

Frankie switched off the TV and shoved the glass of wine behind the sofa, hurriedly straightening the cushions before ushering them in.

They refused her offer of a cup of tea but sat down, side by side, on the sofa. She sat too far away from them on an armchair, trying not to wring her hands, before deciding to drag the chair a bit closer to make the whole thing slightly less formal. They watched her all the while, as if they had already made up their minds that whatever it was that Michael had done, it was his mother's fault.

The male officer took charge. 'So, we want to speak to your son with regard to two incidents; we believe they might be related; end of March time. Easter holidays – round about the 28th or 29th of March or thereabouts?'

Frankie tried to cast her mind back but she couldn't concentrate properly. 'That was before he went away. I can't remember—'

He leant forwards. 'Listen, Mrs Webb. We think your son might have been involved in a very serious assault.'

Frankie sat very still. 'What?'

'A young woman…'

The female officer was watching him warily.

He cleared his throat. 'How shall we put it—'

'A woman was assaulted,' she clarified.

'Yes.' He sat up straighter. 'Allegedly assaulted very seriously,

Mrs Webb,' he added. 'At an address in Iffley.'

Frankie stared, open-mouthed. 'But what makes you think—'

'A sexually motivated attack, we believe.'

Frankie fell silent.

'A white male, apparently,' he continued. 'Dark hair – we haven't got a good description of the face.'

Frankie came to her senses. 'Well, this is just ridiculous.' She looked all around her. 'What on earth makes you think Michael was—'

'Because of the weapon, Mrs Webb.'

Frankie stared, baffled.

'He was carrying a weapon, you see. Some sort of gun, the girl says. Same evening as another one goes missing, as it happens…'

Frankie felt her chest tighten. The air wasn't getting in properly. She tried to sit straighter but she could feel the light shifting, before her eyes, turning everything grey.

'And we think this might be connected to this other incident, you see. Alleged theft of a licensed shotgun – from a Willows Farm.' He checked his notebook. 'Misselden – South Oxfordshire.'

The words dropped like an iron gate between them. And although Frankie could hear what the policeman was saying, she felt as though she was not really there. She tried to cough.

'The residence of a Mr Callum Webb, a farmer.'

Frankie didn't know what to say or do.

And so she said nothing.

'The gentleman's believed to be known to yourself – to your son. That correct, Mrs Webb?'.

'Callum?' Frankie whispered. 'Yes, of course I know him. He's my husband. Well, technically, we're separated.'

'And your son? Can you remember what he was up to that particular evening – end of March?' He glanced at his colleague. 'Bank holiday, wasn't it?'

'Good Friday.' She nodded.

Frankie shook her head. 'He was on a retreat. He's part of a church group. He's very religious, actually, Michael. Do you know St Thomas's? Near Florence Park?'

They exchanged glances. The male officer jotted something down.

'I can't remember the exact place he said they were going…' She trailed off.

And although the female officer was trying to tell her something, while her colleague scribbled away, Frankie couldn't concentrate. All she could see was Callum, all those years before, at the piano. And then Michael, a few weeks before his exams, like a ghost, wrapped in that old yellowed duvet, in Callum's arms.

'Are you alright, Mrs Webb?' The woman's voice was suddenly too loud, as if Frankie were emerging from a dream.

'I'm sorry.' Frankie wiped her eyes. 'It's not Michael.' She felt like she was going to be sick and she tried to breathe more deeply. 'Michael wouldn't hurt…' She didn't know how to finish the thought.

'You look a bit pale, Mrs Webb. Would you like a glass of water?'

'It probably isn't even true. How do you know she's telling the truth?'

'We're not suggesting anyone's telling the truth or not telling the truth at this stage,' the female officer replied gently. 'All we can say is there are extensive injuries. And a witness.'

'Well, it's not Michael,' Frankie said again. 'It can't possibly be. He's a good boy. You don't understand. He's not like that. Honestly.'

The male officer was nodding sympathetically. 'Sometimes even our own family can surprise us, can't they?' He paused a while, glancing surreptitiously at his watch. 'Listen, Mrs Webb. We don't want to take up too much more of your time. But we need to know precisely what your son was doing on that night.'

She shook her head fiercely and clamped her mouth shut. 'It was months ago. I need to go through the calendar and...' She looked around wildly.

'Very well.' He hitched his trousers and stood up, nodding to his colleague. 'In that case, maybe we could start by having a little look round your son's bedroom, for example?'

Frankie stood in the doorway of Michael's room, watching the way they looked all around them. The woman noted the loft panel in the ceiling and silently pointed it out to the other officer with her biro.

The chest of drawers was mainly empty – just Michael's school uniform, in the bottom drawer – and a few jumpers. They patted the clothes down before rifling through the sheet music.

Frankie stood up straighter and checked her watch. 'Is this really necessary?' she asked, coming to her senses. 'Honestly, if you'd met Michael, you'd know this is ridiculous. He tells me off if I so much as kill a wasp. I think there must be some mistake. Have you thought—'

They ignored her and started to talk among themselves.

The woman knelt down and patted the bed, feeling with her hands as she stared into mid-air. 'Could we trouble you for a recent pic of your son, Mrs Webb? A headshot preferably?'

'Yes, of course.' Frankie felt suddenly very tired. How long was this going to take? 'I'll have a look in the box downstairs.'

The female officer peered underneath the bed and reached for something.

'What's this?' She dragged out a case.

'What?' Frankie turned back, angry with them for not believing her – not realising what a good boy she had raised. 'It's his clarinet,' she said coldly.

The woman snapped open the case, disturbing a cloud of dust. She wiped the backs of her hands on her trousers and sat back on her heels.

She smiled up at them in triumph. 'Gotcha.'

They all stared in silent fascination at the case, as if they'd stumbled upon a box of treasure.

'What was that about a wasp, Mrs Webb?'

But still Frankie said nothing.

Because underneath a folded concert programme, instead of the pieces of two clarinets, cradled in grooves of thin velvet that she was expecting to see, what they were looking at was the readily assembled components of what appeared to be some sort of large black gun.

***

It was gone eleven by the time the police eventually left, promising to be back first thing in the morning.

And so Frankie sat on the floor of the living room, with an old Clarks shoebox of photographs that she hadn't looked at in years. She wasn't sure she was strong enough to look through them. But she couldn't bear the thought of talking to anyone either. And there was no way she'd be able to sleep – not after all that. And so, instead, she retrieved her glass of wine from behind the sofa and stayed where she was, looking back at the past, and asking herself over and over how on earth she could have misread the situation so spectacularly.

She picked up a little square photo of John in the shed, feeding a lamb a bottle of milk. The corners were rounded and the colours all muted now with age to a rainbow of sepias. He must have been about two, wearing that little brown duffel coat, with the hood up, a look of elation in his eyes. Behind him, Callum was smiling directly at the camera – impossibly young – just out of frame.

There were hardly any of Michael, she realised, as she reached for a different photo, wiping her eye with the back of her hand. It was one of her on the farm with Ray – her hair – feathered at the sides, with a fringe, which while rather suiting her, wasn't quite *her* somehow. She tucked her hair behind her ear.

And here was another one of her at the farm – in the kitchen – crouching over John, who was playing with Gem as a puppy. Gem could only have been a few weeks old. Frankie was wearing that cream Aran-knit jumper over a long, checked summer dress, unaware that the photo was being taken. She peered more closely at the dress, recognising it, abstractly, as one she had bought before finding out she was pregnant again, realising – with a sudden sour taste in her mouth – that it couldn't have been Gem in that case. It must have been Badger, John's puppy, that Callum had put down.

She shivered and instantly ripped it up, stuffing the pieces back in the box.

And then she heard a noise.

She jumped.

It sounded like someone tapping on the window.

She instinctively ducked down behind the sofa to peer up at the window, before creeping to the front door on hands and knees.

There was no-one there.

But then the front door rattled.

All the blood rushed to her stomach.

'Frances,' someone hissed before the letterbox snapped shut.

She breathed out heavily. 'Michael?' She got up to unlock the door. 'Is that you? What on earth—'

He pushed straight past her and into the house. His skin was uncharacteristically tanned and he was dressed in a faded black tee-shirt and a pair of battered grey cords.

'What are you doing here? The police have just left. What's going on?'

He marched into the living room, checking the windows and closing the curtains.

'I need to stay here, Frances. I think you're in danger.' He held her by the shoulders. His grip was surprisingly strong and she flinched, trying to pull away.

'I might be in danger too. It's Dad.' He hesitated. 'I don't know the full picture but I think he's in real trouble.'

She shook herself free from his grasp and lurched backwards. 'Stop it,' she hissed. 'Stop lying to me.'

He looked shocked.

'This isn't about your dad, is it? You're not in any danger. You're hiding. The police told me everything. I'm not a fool, you know. I'm not taking *any* more of this.'

He didn't say anything.

'All these years. I've given you boys everything. And you just rip it all up.'

He nodded very slowly and raised one hand as if he had to break something to her. 'I know how it must look, Frances, but you've got to listen—'

'No.' She walked over to the front door and opened it wide. '*You* listen for once. I've always been there. Done everything. But that's it now. There's nothing left. How dare you bring a gun into my house?'

His expression was unmoved.

'It's disgusting, Michael. I'm utterly... You should be utterly ashamed of yourself. You can go now. I don't want anything more to do with you.'

He opened his mouth to speak, taking a step towards her.

'No.' She held up her hand and stepped back. 'I don't want to hear it.'

'Right.' He nodded again, reaching out as if to embrace her and then he pushed the door closed and held his hand there to bar her exit.

She jumped as if she'd seen a snake. 'Get out now!' She pushed him away, rattling the door handle in her haste.

'It's not what you think, Frances.'

But his voice was too calm.

'I was trying to protect you. I had this terrible dream.' He reached out for her again.

'Don't touch me.' She shuddered, wrapping her arms around herself, as if she were carrying something precious, close to her heart.

'You've got to believe me. It's not safe for you here. It's Dad. I told you about the cows. He's—'

'It's too late for all this.' She started to cry. 'How could you even *think* of bringing a gun into this house?' she said again.

He looked down at the floor. 'It wasn't like that.'

'I don't care anymore,' she said. 'This is not your home anymore, Michael.'

'Frances, I—'

'No. Shut up. Stop calling me that. I hate it.'

He recoiled as if he'd been stung. 'I understand,' he said eventually, reaching out one more time to embrace her.

But she jumped back. 'No. Go away.' She grew aware that her legs had started to shake and she sensed a swarm of black speckles starting to crowd in on her vision. The photographs lay, in a blur, across the carpet.

'Take care, Frances.'

She heard the door close gently behind him.

Resisting the urge to look out of the window to check he'd gone, she knelt down and started, methodically, to gather up the photographs.

But as she stacked them all up again, as if to physically push all the feelings back into the box, she found her mind, quite involuntarily, wrenched back to that period of her life that she had so neatly packed away for all those years. And she asked herself again how she could have pushed him so far away from her that she hadn't even known what country he was in, let alone the whereabouts of his heart.

And she stopped, letting the pictures fall in a heap on her lap.

She closed her eyes, breathed deeply, and for the first time she allowed herself to go back, to try to remember each detail, in case there was something she had overlooked, right back to the time before Michael came along.

THE BROKEN LINE

September 1998

After taking a shower Frankie changed into her new dress, which was made of stiff pale blue cotton – gathered, pleasingly, at the waist – with very thin navy diagonal stripes, as if they had been drawn on with a biro. She ventured out towards the harbour. There were people everywhere – families – and couples out for dinner, and in the distance she could hear a woman singing.

The street down to the harbour was long and cobbled and the heat seemed incongruous with the darkness, leaving her disoriented. Not really sure what to do, and keen not to draw too much attention to herself, she sat down at the first bar that she came to, by the port, and ordered a beer, already rather hot and self-conscious amidst all the other tanned, unencumbered holidaymakers.

As she waited for her drink, she watched a boat pull in, its light catching high on the clifftops, illuminating a church tower and a crescent of white houses that made the island look as though it were smiling. And as she looked across the curve of the bay, she noticed fairy lights zigzagging between the curling seafront tavernas.

She looked around her. Everyone seemed to be laughing. The family at the table next to her were eating the most delicious-looking food – little pastries and stuffed peppers. The waiter appeared to be bringing an endless stream of dishes. And although Frankie pretended to read the menu, she couldn't take her eyes off their table to see what was coming next.

When the waiter asked her if she'd made up her mind, she said she'd like a selection of little dishes, please, like the ones they were having over there, she explained, pointing discreetly.

'The family platter. Of course, Madam.'

She had only meant a little taster of each, she tried to explain, mortified, as he started to bring the food. But he ignored her protests. She glanced furtively around, certain everyone would notice her ordering far too much food for one person as he brought tiny whitebait, soft calamari drenched in lemon, tomatoes still warm from the vine, hunks of salty feta and glistening red onion, enormous black olives, and vine leaves stuffed with warm rice and tender minced lamb. Then came the tray of little goat's cheese pastries, slow-baked aubergines, soft white garlicky beans in tomatoes sprinkled with oregano, and salty courgette fritters. She thought she was going to explode as she reached for the warm, hard-crusted bread to mop up the last of the tzatziki.

Her eyes were woozy from the carafe of sharp white wine that the waiter had insisted on bringing her and the mild aniseed aftertaste of the home-made ouzo which she would never have touched – along with the watermelon – had they not been on the house.

Afterwards, she felt sure she wouldn't be able to move a muscle. But for once, she didn't care. Instead, she sat back in her chair and smiled at all life passing, in pure, slow pleasure, around her, the guide book unopened on the chair beside her.

And the best bit about it all was that no-one paid her the slightest bit of attention. And although she was quite aware that if anyone had been watching her, they would have realised that she looked absolutely idiotic, she couldn't stop smiling.

May 1978

It was early summer – the end of May. John had just turned three and Frankie was ten weeks pregnant. It had been raining incessantly for weeks.

Although she was keen to start telling people about the new baby, she didn't dare talk about it too much because Callum was so preoccupied. The lower fields were partly flooded and the soil had been too wet for the tractors, throwing everything off kilter. On top of that, Lulu, his collie, was out of action until her litter arrived a few weeks later. And Ray's dog, whom Callum nicknamed Snail to wind the other man up, was proving useless without Lulu out ahead.

Frankie remembered how it started – just a couple of specks of blood in her pyjamas.

She'd tried to think nothing of it as she gave John some more toast and cleared away the breakfast things. He wanted to go outside but it was still raining so she persuaded him to do some playdough for a bit, just until it eased off, while she cleaned up the mess in the utility room from where the chickens had got in.

There was a third speck, though, when she went up to get dressed, so she called the surgery, just to be on the safe side.

Bill Edwards agreed to see her immediately if things got any worse, and advised her on the phone to monitor it at home, but to come in – and to bring some towels with her – if the bleeding got very heavy, which it did unfortunately, she realised, late in the afternoon, as she lay down numb on her bed, listening for John still splashing in the yard, feeling the sensation of her future leaking out of her.

And to remember to keep any large clots.

The rain was getting heavier. And before getting up to go into the bathroom she watched the water wriggling down the thick window panes, the light catching, so that its shadow danced on the wall, like the tail of a fish writhing in a net.

She knelt down to get some pads from the bathroom cupboard to get ready to go into the surgery, worrying about how to get hold of Callum so she could leave John at home rather than take him with her. She stood up too quickly, aghast to feel a strange sensation – her movement unbalanced – as if she had stepped off a boat.

She looked down and gasped. Something had come out of her – dark purple – a mesh of blood. It hung between her legs.

She felt a wave of nausea.

There was a bang on the door.

She grabbed the basin to stop herself falling.

'Mummy! Look what I've found.'

She caught the clot on a wad of toilet paper, uncertain what to do with it.

And with shaking hands she stared at it until she noticed a tiny bubble inside, no bigger than a grain of rice, cradling what looked like a minuscule newt, or a treble clef, with its tail curled in.

John started to bang louder.

'Just a minute, John,' she said, her voice wobbling, unfamiliar.

And from nowhere she saw the face of that Greek woman on their honeymoon – the half-smile as she had turned away.

She sat on the edge of the bath, staring out the window, until the banging and the screaming was so loud that she could endure it no longer. She pulled down the blinds. Through the coarse beige fabric she could just make out the outline of the cowshed where someone was shovelling, the grating sound of the spade on cement reminding her of a gravedigger accidentally encountering stone.

The light had started to change.

And she looked down one last time at that little thing – knowing it – like she knew her own reflection – to have been her second child.

Afterwards she lay back down on the bed and stared at the wall, one ear to the half-light, listening to the rain.

From the doorway, John watched her. He had taken his coat off but was still in his wellies, clutching a miniature brown teddy bear with limbs that only danced when he was there. In the other hand, he was carrying a grey and white feather from a pigeon.

'John, come and lie down.'

He took off his boots and climbed up beside her. He was warm and his little hands were stained blue from the dried-out playdough; she could smell it – somewhere between suntan lotion and marzipan. And she held him close.

He started singing very softly. *'The farmer's in his den. The farmer's in his den. Ee-ay-ah-di-oh, the farmer's in his den.'*

And after a couple of lines, she joined in with him, following his lead, as he rotated the legs of the teddy bear, mixing and blurring the lines as he went, so it wasn't clear, by the time they reached bone, what it was that the farmer had even wanted – let alone the wife or the child.

She watched the reflection of the rain forge new shapes on the wall, feeling the blood giving way to air, marking – with each pain – the rhythm of the loss, like a pulse felt only by the silence and succession of its beat.

***

She hadn't been able to talk to Callum about any of it. He was worried about her; she could tell. But she couldn't articulate why it had upset her so much. It had only been a few weeks. She'd barely had time to acknowledge she was even pregnant.

He kept pushing, though.

'No,' she had snapped one evening, shoving the basket of clean laundry off the bed so that the sheets fell, in a formless mound, on the carpet. 'I don't have to square up to anything. You don't know anything.'

He tried to hold her but she clenched all her muscles so that he shrank back. 'It's worse otherwise,' he said. 'Because it's still there – it doesn't go anywhere – it just keeps piling up.'

As the days passed, she could tell that John sensed something had changed, too. He started refusing to go to sleep at night, crying for hours as she sat exhausted by his side.

When Lulu had her puppies, he wanted to keep the little one. They'd named him Badger because of the white patches on his eyes and front paws. The others sold quickly but Badger was too jumpy and Frankie wasn't sure, privately, if anyone was going to take him. But she couldn't cope with another dog at that time – not while John was still in nappies – and she told John that Daddy had already explained why they couldn't keep the puppies. They'd have to let Badger go and live with another family.

But it escalated.

And she had had days of John screaming. In the end, she couldn't take it anymore and gave in, telling him he could keep Badger, provided he promised to help her take care of him.

But Callum was furious. 'I already told him we couldn't

keep it,' he said that evening as she mopped the kitchen floor – for the fifth time that day – in the place where John had been playing with the puppies.

Her back ached. She hadn't eaten anything since breakfast.

And she felt a strong urge to scream in Callum's face.

'He has to learn. You need to be firmer with him, not all this molly-coddling.'

'Oh, really?' She stared him straight in the eye. 'Well, you know what? Here you go.' She thrust the mop into his hand. 'Why don't *you* teach him? Because I'm out of here.'

And then she marched up the stairs to John's room to pull the suitcase out from under the spare bed. John was standing in his cot, still screaming.

'It's okay, John. Mummy's here,' she said, crouched on the floor as she pulled all his clothes out of the chest of drawers.

She deliberately took no notice when she heard Callum follow her upstairs. But she sensed him, out of the corner of her eye, in the door frame, blocking her next move.

September 1998

That week Frankie spent the days swimming. The physiotherapist had told her that swimming would be good for the leg – and she had obviously been proved right about that on top of everything else. Frankie could feel the muscles strengthening by the day.

Her skin turned darker than it had ever been – her back and shoulders so tanned that from behind she would have been unrecognisable.

And as she swam, her arms and legs co-operating so smoothly it was as if they belonged to someone else, she set her mind free to dream. She thought of all the things that she loved to do but never gave herself enough time for. And all the time she wasted on things that seemed only to squash her life and her soul – her thoughts momentarily interrupted by the realisation that she had forgotten all about looking into those spa alternatives for Olivia that she had promised. She'd do it when she got back, she reasoned, pushing it out of her mind and concentrating instead on why it had been so many years since she last swam in the sea, for example.

Why was that?

She pictured that cottage she'd seen from the window of the B&B in New Quay after she had left Callum for the first time – up high, in a wild garden trailing down to the sea.

And she resolved, as she headed further and further each day from the shore, that when she got back home, she would live a very different sort of life – be a very different sort of person, in short, from the one she'd been settling for all these years. The sort of person who actually lives in an impractical place like that; runs their own café; has a garden overlooking the sea; who goes swimming in the sea, for that matter. She stared back at the sun, through the reflection on the water's surface. Yes, every day, she felt like saying, squinting at its scornful glare.

Especially in winter, she decided.

She knew the sort. She'd watched them in those weeks in New Quay. She used to spend hours feeding Michael on a bench that overlooked the beach, while John traipsed along the sand, oblivious to the cold, dragging buckets full of pebbles and trailing seaweed that would defrost into a slimy pulp by the time they got back to their room. It was older women, always, in racer-back navy swimming costumes and swimming caps. The way they waded into the sea, their backs to the huddles of dog-walkers throwing sticks. Not only as if they didn't feel the cold, but as if they didn't inhabit the same world as everyone else. And although she had admired them, she hadn't properly understood them.

Until now, that is.

Now she realised that it was a sort of freedom they were choosing to exercise. To step aside from the pack. To just be who they wanted to be. And do exactly as they liked – almost in defiance of the very elements themselves.

June 1978

Although she had wanted to go to John, who had stopped crying and was standing up now in his cot, reaching for her, Frankie found that she was entirely unable to move. It was as if all the bones in her back and legs had been broken by the incident, one by one by one.

She lay on the spare bed. Everything ached. Everything was bruised. But she didn't care now, and besides, the pain was more bearable, she found, when she was lying down.

John was whimpering. He needed her to pick him up. She knew she should. But she couldn't bear to touch him. Couldn't bear to be with anyone. She pulled the duvet up tight under her chin and let her legs rest – they were still shaking from the position she had been holding, without realising.

She closed her eyes but all she could see was John's expression and she wondered if she would ever be able to sleep again without seeing that little face.

'It's okay,' she whispered, the tears pressing now beneath the surface of her skin like a new bruise building.

She hauled her fragile broken body to an upright position and hobbled over to pick John out of his cot, as if someone else were directing her limbs. The half-packed suitcase lay against the chest of drawers where she had left it, with John's clothes in a heap on the floor.

She lay John down in the bed alongside her. He clung so hard to her arms that she felt they could ache no more.

But she tucked his head beneath her chin so that he wouldn't see her tears. She stroked his back. 'Don't cry, Mummy's here.'

That night she lay awake for hours. And eventually, when her body could withstand it no longer, she fell into a sudden, fragile, sleep.

In her dream, the room was on fire. She needed to get out. But her legs were broken. John was with her and all the bedding was on fire. She tried to flap it and crush the air out of it but it was getting hotter and hotter. She crawled to the bathroom for water but when she got there she realised John was already in the bath, lying beneath the surface of the water, and when she tried to lift him out, the water was ice-cold. But even though his body was stiff and blue, his eyes were wide open, and he was staring up at her.

At five the next morning Frankie was awoken by the sound of Callum going down to the kitchen. Although she felt as if she'd been awake all night, she must have drifted off at some point. She stayed where she was, in the spare bed, the horror of the previous evening unfolding in a loop like a sequence from a film that has got stuck. John was still asleep beside her. When she looked down at him, she had a brief memory of the dream and grabbed him to check he was breathing.

She knew she had to get out of there but wasn't sure where to begin anymore. Her back ached as if she had been pummelled all over. And everything seemed so pointless. Where would they even go? How would she carry their things?

It was stupid.

And then something else struck her.

It suddenly occurred to her that Callum hadn't used a condom. And she wondered why she hadn't thought of that while it was happening. She touched the tops of her legs, gingerly, to try and start to work out the extent of the damage but a pain shot through her and she had to clench her mouth shut to stop herself crying out and waking John.

But the thought wouldn't go away. With a sense of trepidation, she patted her stomach. Her skin seemed too tender where the bruising was starting to emerge.

She tried to steady her breathing. She had to stay calm. Everything was okay, she told herself. She'd go to the doctor. She could get a test.

Her face stung as she pictured Dr Edwards's expression. No, she couldn't go back to him so soon. She tried to remember when her period had been – a couple of weeks ago, wasn't it? No, more, she realised. But things hadn't been the same since the miscarriage. And Dr Edwards had warned her that it could take time to regulate.

But she just couldn't remember and her mind was all tangled up.

John stirred.

She couldn't let John see her like this. She needed to clean herself up.

She managed to heave her burning body into the bathroom. She shuddered as she reached down to put the bath plug in and saw, as if it belonged to someone else, that there was a little clump of her hair, caught in the plug hole, where Callum had held her by the back of the neck.

Her breathing quickened and she sat down heavily on the floor with her back against the bath. Her hands and feet were cold and everything hurt. She closed her eyes, feeling her vision dissolve in the damp grey steam, uncertain she would ever be able to get up again.

*

She was right. There had been no real point worrying about it. There really was nowhere to go. Callum must have taken the Land Rover up to Conway's field and there was no sign of the van, she had realised, with a dull sense of despair as she felt her future trickle away, like sand, through her fingers.

Maybe it was easier to just stay where they were. She looked over at John in front of the TV, still in his pyjamas, watching *Rainbow*; they'd zipped up Zippy's mouth but John wasn't laughing that day. She sat on the stairs. Maybe she could go to the doctor the next day, she reasoned blindly.

But by the afternoon she was distraught. She lay on the sofa, waiting for the surgery to return her call, as John climbed on her. Although the pain was unbearable it was a fraction more comfortable than attempting to stand up or walk, which simply made her feel as though all her insides were in danger of falling straight out. She wanted to sleep but her eyes wouldn't relax, and besides, that wasn't an option because John wanted to play.

'Piggyback, Mummy,' he whined, as she lay there like a bag of cement.

'No, John,' she snapped, causing his little face to fold in despair. But she couldn't bring herself to comfort him. And she wondered, in that moment, if there would ever be a time again when the whole world would just leave her alone.

When Nina, the receptionist from the surgery, eventually rang back, it seemed to take Frankie hours to crawl to the phone. They'd made an appointment for ten past three the following afternoon with Bill Edwards.

She held her breath, trying not to burst into tears or be rude to Nina, knowing how much she had hated dealing with angry patients herself. 'I don't suppose there's anything with any of the others, is there?' There was a loud clattering sound from the other room. And then a strong silence. She looked around wildly. Where was John?

'Sorry, Frankie, it's completely chock-a-block for some reason this week. Miles is still off, so there's a huge backlog there and it's baby clinic, obviously, tomorrow afternoon, so that's all the nurses out, too.'

John started to scream at the top of his voice.

'Just a minute, John,' Frankie called to him, her hand over the receiver.

'Bill and Helen are both fully booked today. So would you—'

'No.' Frankie could barely hear Nina over John's screams. 'I'll come tomorrow,' she said, hobbling to comfort John, and wondering all the while how she could possibly get anywhere in this condition.

Even though she waited up for him that night, Callum didn't come back in. She went to bed in the end, leaving his dinner under an upturned casserole dish on the kitchen table, deciding to sleep a second night in the spare bed in John's room.

The next day she woke up with an extreme sense of foreboding and realised, as she ventured into their bedroom, that Callum had left the house again without waking her. As she pulled on some clothes, she sensed all that hope she had dared to let herself feel, at the prospect of a new start, seep out of her body, leaving only a dull, heavy nothingness, like wet clay, in its place, as she concentrated instead on what on earth she was going to say to Dr Edwards.

Dr Edwards was running late. By half-past three, John had not only eaten the entire packet of Digestives that she'd brought with her but had also – despite complaining of a tummy ache

– started to work his way through a bag of dried apricots. He'd shown no interest in the colouring book nor in her half-hearted suggestion of a game of I Spy and had started to whine loudly that he wanted to go home.

The waiting room was full of mothers and babies and she could sense them staring at her – seeing all too clearly that she had no idea what she was doing as she sat there, pretending to read an ancient copy of *Woman's Own*. When she accidentally caught Nina's eye, watching her from behind the desk, Frankie felt as though she might burst into tears.

When John ran off towards the examining rooms, she jumped up, face flaming, and hauled him, yelling in protest, back to where they'd been sitting. But the more she tried to gently persuade him to calm down, the louder he howled, until he broke free of her grasp altogether and threw himself face-first to the floor, where he continued to scream, all the while kicking the chair legs of the woman sitting next to Frankie, until her name was finally called.

Dr Edwards greeted her with a beaming smile, his small darting eyes flickering over her, seemingly oblivious to her furious purple child. 'Frankie, so nice to see you. You're looking well. As you can see, things have completely gone to pieces since you abandoned us!'

She pretended to laugh. 'Come on, John,' she whispered. 'We're nearly finished now. Let's see if the doctor's got any of those nice Dennis the Menace stickers.'

John instantly stopped crying. 'Okay,' he said.

'How are things, Frankie? How's Callum?'

'Great, thanks, Bill. Yes, we're all fine, thanks.' Feigning a smile, she half-pushed John into the room in front of her, like a shield. 'Keeping busy with this little tearaway...' She trailed off, wondering how she was going to broach the subject.

'Good, good.' He scribbled something down and patted his damp grey hair at the sides to smooth it into place. 'And how's the farm?' He spun round to face her.

'No, it's all fine, thanks – pretty chaotic, as always, but we're holding up, just about…' She could feel her cheeks wobbling and she reached for a tissue, pretending to wipe John's mouth. He cried out in annoyance. 'How are you? Angie well?'

John was still whining. She squeezed his hand to reassure him that he wouldn't have to wait much longer. Her palms were sweating.

'Good, good. So, what can we do for you today, then?'

'Well, it's a bit embarrassing actually.' She was horrified to feel herself start to blush. 'But I need to get… er… a pregnancy test,' she mouthed, patting John on the head as she attempted to gently cover his ears. She laughed awkwardly as Dr Edwards raised his eyebrows and placed a finger to his lips. 'Many congratulations to you both,' he whispered.

She shrank back. 'It's a bit of a surprise, actually. And it's far too early to test. But I wanted to be on the front foot.' She looked up at the clock, wondering how long they would have to sit there before she screamed out loud.

He busied himself on his computer, suddenly serious. 'Right, right, and can I ask how your contraception choices are working more generally, Mrs Webb? What is it that you are using, as a rule, these days?'

He turned and stared right at her. She noticed the muscle in his cheek twitch.

Her face ached from all that smiling and she resisted a strong urge to punch him on the nose. 'Just condoms,' she said quickly, evading his gaze and feeling her face getting hotter and hotter, the longer he stared at her, nodding and scribbling, scribbling and nodding.

John was watching her carefully.

'And would you like to consider any alternatives to—'

'No thanks,' she added – her voice coming out too high. 'We're fine actually. It's still early days, as I said. I'd be very grateful, Bill – not that you would of course – but if you didn't mention it to—'

'Of course, of course. No problem,' he added solemnly.

She laughed awkwardly.

'Here we go.' Ignoring Frankie, he signed his name with a flourish, then shook her by the hand, holding on for a moment too long.

'Great. Thanks.' She stood up too fast – a shooting pain down one leg – and snatched the prescription with such haste that it almost ripped.

She hurried home and hid the test immediately at the back of her wardrobe.

***

The weeks passed; the pregnancy test was negative, when it came to it, and eventually things ground back to normal.

The only difference was that Frankie found she had lost all interest in everything. It was enough to just get through the day without giving in to the overwhelming sense of dread that hung over her like fog. Although she found it increasingly difficult to fall asleep each night, from the moment she opened her eyes in the morning, she would count down the hours until she could go back to bed.

She lost her appetite, too; tea tasted like soap; and everything seemed to be shrouded in a rotten sweet smell – like decaying lilies – leaving her nauseous at the mere thought of food. She developed an unpleasant metallic taste in her mouth, too, that no amount of antiseptic mouthwash seemed to shift. The face that greeted her in the mirror each morning was that of her mother: pale, drawn and guarded.

And so, after two months had passed and her periods still hadn't returned, she simply hadn't known who to turn to.

In the end she ducked into the local pharmacy, with John, to get another test, before hovering, against all better judgement, in the public toilet in town to find out. It was surprisingly cold in there and it stank like silage. She noticed, stepping over pools of stagnant water, that all the locks were broken and that there was no toilet paper. As she stood in the cubicle in her raincoat, stick in hand, with John squashed up against her, begging her to tell him a story, she stared at her watch, urging the time to pass more quickly, as she concentrated on trying not to be sick.

She almost didn't need to see the second line start to emerge, as if from a great distance, to tell her what she realised she had always known, that there was something rotten, still, inside her. Something that wasn't meant to be there.

But she waited nevertheless – entirely unable to move.

Not even when the second line was as strong as the first.

She wasn't sure what she was waiting for anymore.

But she didn't know, either, what she was supposed to do next.

She felt completely empty.

She stared at the grey metal door. Someone had taped up a leaflet warning about the risk of sharing needles; the same one from the surgery, she realised dispassionately. The corner, with the phone number, had been torn off.

It felt as if she had been caught – as if, having carefully hidden away her real self all these years, someone had finally caught up with her, spotted her cowering, and dragged her out by the hair into the middle of the road to leave her there, on display, so that everyone could finally see that dark empty badness deep inside her that was growing, like mould – thickening, now – so that before long it would engulf everything and snuff out her soul.

***

And so the weeks went by, bleeding slowly into months.

Frankie dutifully registered the pregnancy with Dr Edwards and went to see the midwives periodically at the hospital, who assured her, despite her concerns to the contrary, that Baby was growing nicely and was expected to arrive in the middle of March.

She couldn't bring herself to look at the screen when it was time for the ultrasound. She told them she was superstitious and that she didn't want to know if it was a boy or a girl, staring so hard, instead, at the tessellating ceiling tiles that they looked as though they were collapsing in on her. Because the truth was that she couldn't bear to confront the evidence that, in spite of everything she had tried, there was something bad inside her that refused to leave her alone. And she knew that it couldn't possibly come to any good.

'Oh, look,' the sonographer chuckled to the nurse. 'We've got a thumb sucker.'

Frankie pretended to smile as she closed her eyes to stop them leaking. Although her hands and feet were cold her face felt hot and the bones of her skull too tight. She wondered if she should tell them how much pain she was in and whether there was something she could take for it. To make it all go away.

But she said nothing and lay very still, aware of the sensation of the weight of the baby and the uterus pressing down into her back, as if to physically block her airways of all hope as she imagined the darkness growing bigger inside her and tried to silence the words of the palm-reader on her honeymoon that coursed through her head like a prayer to the devil.

Instead, she did as she was told, and behaved, in short, like a proper mother. She stocked up on nappies and Napisan and Milupa as early as January and dusted off all John's old baby accoutrements that they had stored away in the barn for the best part of the last year – the highchair, plastic bath, that little bouncing baby seat and a suitcase of carefully pressed off-white babygros and bibs – not to mention pile after lovingly folded pile of muslins and towelling nappies. Because she had always told herself, back then, that when it came down to it, there was nothing else she could really do.

But as she sat, all those years later, sifting through those old photographs, she wondered again whether things would have turned out differently had *she* done things differently – perhaps got away sooner, for example – or whether life was merely panning out in its own stubbornly inevitable way, just as it always did – just as the lines had predicted.

She looked down at the picture in her hand. It was of Michael, aged four, on his first day at school. He was standing on the doorstep, staring up at her – the eyes too solemn and too knowing to belong, rightfully, to any child. And she realised she could see the man in that face, even then – the man he would become – with no whisper of a smile to soften the thudding realisation that the truth had been right in front of her all these years. She had just been too stubborn to accept it.

It was simple.

Case closed.

His father's son.

September 1998

After her swim each day, when Frankie returned to the hot sand, she detected a new vitality – a lightness of heart – that seemed to pump through her entire body. And a lightness of foot to match, almost as if to spite her aching limbs from so many hours out at sea, so that she sprang back to the shade of the tamarisk like a mountain goat.

In the evenings she ate early, armed with a notebook – before the tavernas got busy – filling her stomach with as much of that delicious food as she could squeeze in, knowing it would set her up for the next day's swim, and treating it as research, more than anything, for the sort of dishes she would serve in her own café, making plans – with diagrams – for her return, before retreating to her dark cool bed where she slept deeply for ten hours at a time.

September 1997

In the end, Michael didn't only pass his exams, he scored the highest it was possible to score on every single paper.

The examination board even wrote to him and to his head teacher on results day to personally congratulate him even though he was long gone by then.

Frankie wasn't sure he'd ever even found out what his grades had been, let alone read that letter, which she opened herself eventually, one morning a few weeks after that visit from the police. But it didn't seem to matter in the way it once had and she resealed the envelope, propping it up on his chest of drawers where she had first placed it, on top of his stack of sheet music that had lain, ignored, for all that time, along with what she had so naively believed to have been his clarinet under the bed. And when she came to pack up his room the following year, she couldn't bring herself to throw the letter away.

Frankie pestered the police continuously in the weeks that followed their visit. But whenever she called to ask for an update, quoting the reference number they had given her, she got the same response. They thanked her for her call but explained that they were unable to comment on an ongoing investigation.

She also phoned Monira, at the homeless shelter, a couple of times, asking if she'd heard from Michael. But Monira said she hadn't seen Michael in months and felt awful about some misunderstanding they had had. She had been trying to get hold of him herself, as it happened, in case he was interested in a job that was coming up and she asked Frankie to let her know if she heard from him.

Frankie scoured the *Oxford Times* for clues, too, lingering occasionally under her horoscope, on the lonely hearts column, taken aback by the sheer volume of elderly gentlemen in the area who wanted to embark on long walks with significantly younger women – blonde and brunette in equal measure, it seemed – provided they were trim, slim or petite with a good sense of humour and no trace of cigarette smoke. And – not unlike those same gentlemen – she found herself wondering, stony-faced, as she got ready for bed each night, where all these hilarious miniature women were, limbering up to walk off the best years of their life in the company of so many indescribably ghastly old men.

But her search for news of Michael's whereabouts proved fruitless: there was never any mention of him.

Although she had no idea where he was, she started to write to Michael, too. Several times. To see if she could work out what she wanted to say. She found it hard to get the words right, though.

I appreciate I may not understand all the details yet, Michael, but let's just say I am extremely upset by what the police have told me so far, and I'm afraid you caught me at rather a bad moment when you turned up that night before the news had even sunk in. Of course, I need to hear from you exactly what's happened but I'm sure you'll agree it would be so much better to be able to talk about all this on the phone or in person. I hope you might explain it all a bit more clearly for me. It's very important, Michael.

She frowned and underlined '*very important*' twice, as she read it back to herself aloud, crossing out the two previous lines.

She changed tack.

Perhaps we could have a little chat on the phone when you have a moment?

She bit her lip and looked out the window. It reminded her of all those letters she used to write to her mum.

You know you can always talk to me.

She shook her head. The words weren't right.

Whatever you've done, I'm still your mum and I'll always be there for you.

Love, Mum.

She paused, staring at the words as they blurred. She tutted to herself and wiped her eye, dabbing the smudged ink with her sleeve, accidentally blotting out the Mum even further, so that the love was no longer visible anymore either.

She crossed out the whole of the last bit and sat up straighter, reminding herself of the expression the policeman had used: 'sexually motivated'.

And then she crossed the rest of it out, too, before ripping it up and starting again on a fresh sheet, a little more business-like and to the point, this time. 'With love, from Frankie.'

But of course, she had nowhere to send it.

***

Weeks passed and then months and still there was no word from Michael.

She could think of nothing else. Every time the phone rang, she raced to answer it, longing more than anything to hear his voice.

Christmas came and went – her first ever alone. And although John said that Brian and Susanna Whitaker had made it clear that they had loads of space down in Winchester and that Frankie was more than welcome to spend it with them – apparently, they *hated* the thought of her all alone – she reassured John that she was, in fact, very much looking forward to a bit of peace and quiet for a change, not to mention an early night.

Because she couldn't explain – not to John, not to anyone – how much she missed him – how she missed having the boys at home – or how she secretly longed to see Michael, whatever he had done, even though she knew it was irrational.

And in the end, it started to dawn on her that perhaps Michael was well and truly gone from her life.

And so, when the phone rang a few weeks later, on her birthday – one Saturday afternoon in February – she didn't think for a moment that it would be Michael.

She had been out the night before for a lacklustre meal with the girls from the surgery. She'd been working extra shifts, partly to save a bit of cash to help John and Olivia with the wedding, but mainly to avoid being in the house for any longer than she could bear, and she hadn't wanted to go out at all but they'd insisted, telling her it was the least they could do after the week she had had. Said it would do her the world of good; they were going straight after work; it was their shout and they weren't taking no for an answer.

It wasn't just the events of recent months, nor especially the act of turning forty-five in itself; the truth was that she hadn't seen much to celebrate for many years. She'd spent so long feeling afraid of something. And even when she reminded herself that Callum was as good as gone now – she hadn't seen him in the best part of ten months – instead of feeling glad and light she felt an even greater weight on her spirit than ever. Although the anxiety had gone, in its place lay a great crushing flatness, only mildly tempered, on occasion, with a drifting guilt for all those years gone to waste. She had thrown away all those precious years, waiting to be alone, and when it came to it, she realised she had forgotten to make any plans for the afterwards bit.

And all she wanted – more than anything – was to have the boys back.

For the first time in her life, she hated silence.

It greeted her, like a prison guard, when she got up every morning. And she came to dread the weekends, finding that sometimes a whole day or two could pass without speaking to anyone at all. It felt like lying under a great mattress that had been dunked in a canal.

And as she looked around the cavernous restaurant, stuffed full of young couples and commuters and children crayoning on to paper placemats, she realised that she was the oldest person in there. Men in stripy tee-shirts with Italian pseudonyms cooked pizza behind her and the noise from the stacking of plates and screeching of cappuccino machines made it difficult to follow the conversation around the table. Debbie, the other receptionist, was aggressively refilling wine glasses as she attempted to persuade Frankie to go on a blind date with a man called Nick – a friend of her brother-in-law whom she had met in January on a skiing holiday in Chamonix and who had recently got divorced.

'He's Irish – drop-dead gorgeous,' she kept saying with great seriousness as she swept her purply-black hair from her eyes. 'Cross between Pierce Brosnan and Billy Baldwin. Lives in Hemel Hempstead. Made a lot of money in self-storage, by all accounts. Got teenage kids. But they're with the mum, I think. Absolutely loaded, evidently.'

'Right.' Frankie nodded politely, her forehead heavy from the woody white wine.

'Honestly, I had half a mind to ditch Simon right there

and then on the slopes when Gail mentioned Nick was still single.' She cackled and a fine spray of spit landed like mist on Frankie's cheekbone. She waited until Debbie looked the other way before wiping it off.

'And I'm there thinking: how is *he* still single? And I'm racking my brains for any single ladies and first thought comes into my head, well – obviously – what about Frankie?'

'Right,' Frankie said again, accidentally catching sight of her reflection in the mirror in the distance. Her hair was frizzy from the rain. She tucked it behind her ear, feeling her face stiffen. She looked down at the table.

'So, I said to him, "Well, what's your type, Nick?" And I think he'd really like you, actually, Frankie. I hope you don't mind but I did casually, you know, kind of drop you into the conversation...'

Frankie didn't say anything.

'And I explained that you've got grown-up kids, too, and he said that to be honest everyone's got baggage when you're dating second time round.'

'Did he?' Frankie said evenly.

'Yes, and he said that wasn't really a deal-breaker for him. Said he's kind of interested in being with someone at a similar stage of life, actually, this time. So long as they, you know, take care of themselves.'

Frankie's jaw stiffened. 'Rather than taking care of everyone else, you mean?'

Debbie didn't seem to hear her. 'And I said, well, I've got a colleague, Frankie, who's absolutely lovely who'd be *right* up your street by the sounds of it. She's ever so nice, I said, and a nice figure too – you know, lovely and slim.'

Frankie frowned. 'I'm not sure he sounds like *my* type, actually. Thanks, though.'

'What?' Debbie raised her eyebrows and gave a snort. 'What do you mean he's not your type? He's everyone's type.'

'I'm sure he's perfectly nice but I'm not sure I want to spend my time with someone who thinks the most important quality in a woman is how little space she takes up.'

Debbie stared at her, open-mouthed. 'What are you on about? You know what, Frankie. I like you a lot. You know I do. And please don't take this the wrong way but you could do with lightening up a bit. I reckon you'd be a lot more fun.' And then she had turned, rather pointedly, to her left, with her back to Frankie so Frankie could no longer hear any of the conversation.

And so she stayed silent, letting everyone else decide to stretch the evening out too long, moving on to a bar that had just opened on the Iffley Road that was not much bigger than a wardrobe, painted black inside, with expensive cocktails, deafening house music and lime-green plastic stools that were too high and which spun when Frankie tried to sit down so that she accidentally knocked into the floor-to-ceiling mirror that loomed over her as if to make itself seem bigger than it truly was.

By the time they left it was past midnight. It was still raining and no buses passed so Frankie had to walk all the way home. When she got back, she felt flattened and acutely aware that it had been far too long since she had enjoyed anything.

Unable to sleep and fed up with the last two crossword clues, she found herself rereading an update on the BSE inquiry; there was a photo of the boy who had died; he reminded her so much of Michael; and a quote from his mother – how she'd known something was wrong but the doctors hadn't listened.

Frankie shuddered, her mind racing.

She turned to the back of the paper for something lighter, scanning the horoscopes and the small ads out of habit, half an eye open for that artist who had caught her fancy, if she ignored the reference to walks, that is. Idly noting the PO Box number, her eyes flitting over the rest of the page, she wondered who all those other Pisceans were who were able to abandon everything at the drop of a hat and actually capitalise on the moon being in Jupiter, for once, and just *go* on a bloody holiday.

Devastatingly attractive artist, M (wrong side of 43) seeks F for walks, talks, boat trips and other outdoor acts of love. Must have enormous a) imagination and b) heart.

She thought back to that thing Debbie had said.

And as she lay there in the dark, she mentally composed a letter to that man in the paper. She couldn't possibly use her real name, in case anyone found out. And Frances was far too old-fashioned and conventional. She needed something completely different — more artistic, for a start. Maybe a Phoebe or a Jasmine or something? She squinted, imagining Jasmine, barefoot, in a flowing smock dress, brimming with compassion, her ringleted black hair crowned with primroses.

She read it again and then she ripped it out and placed it, as a marker, in the final Ripley book that she'd had to order in from the library, lingering on the opening paragraph.

No. He probably wouldn't even reply.

She didn't need to give any personal information away — she could provide her phone number and then just backtrack — pretend it was a wrong number or something if she changed her mind — or if the artist thing was just a cover and he turned out, unbeknownst to his neighbours for all those years, to have been a psychotic stalker of vulnerable middle-aged women, storing their enormous butchered hearts in his freezer in the first-floor flat of a 1930s semi in Hillingdon.

Yes, on balance, if he didn't reply, nothing lost.

And if he did reply, well, she'd just leave that bit to fate.

And not only that; she determined to contact Southey and Sons – first thing in the morning – to instruct them to issue the divorce proceedings that had been on hold for nineteen years too long.

September 1998

On the last day of her holiday, she swam further out than she'd ever been, towards a tiny uninhabited island, more like a giant rock, really, that sat about three miles from the shore, she calculated, exactly halfway between the two ends of the beach.

She had swum near the rock before, of course, but it always looked closer than it actually was. And she had always lost her nerve in the end.

But that day she persevered. There was a bird perched on the top and she wanted to see what it was. She knew it was probably foolish; the sun was getting hotter overhead and it must be well past one o'clock now, she realised, glancing over her shoulder and feeling a little uneasy about how long it would take her to get back. When she got closer to the sea bird, she decided it must be a type of cormorant. It was standing very still with its wings outstretched, as if it were sunbathing, and the way the sunlight brushed the top of its head gave the illusion that it were coated in suntan oil. It didn't move as she approached.

Although the rock was covered in thick layers of seaweed on most of one side, it looked unwelcomingly sharp underneath. But she found, as she swam around, that there were a few places where it was worn smooth enough to test a foot.

She clambered on, gripping tightly to the surface. She cut her hand and cried out, not loudly, but it was enough to send the cormorant on its way. She clung on and managed to find a patch that looked soft enough to sit on.

She accidentally snagged her bikini bottoms as she sat down and noticed a little rip on one side. She quickly looked all around her to check no-one had seen, before realising how ridiculous she was. And there, in the middle of the ocean, she laughed out loud. 'Frances Webb, you are a right idiot sometimes.'

She gazed at the beach, the people no bigger than insects, while up on the cliff miniature figures crawled amidst the brown gorse and wild purple heather. And all at once she pictured that garden again in New Quay – the one she had been thinking about all week – terraced, on different levels, and wildly overgrown as if it had accidentally dropped something over the cliff and were stretching down to the coastline to retrieve it.

Yes, she thought as she reclined, closing her eyes and adjusting position to avoid a jagged ledge that was scratching her spine. That was the kind of place she was after.

Behind her eyelids orange and red shapes collided and bloomed like geraniums. And she thought again about Omar and wondered whether he would like it there. She was almost afraid to admit it but she wanted him to see the real her, next time, and although she couldn't be sure he'd still like her she knew now that she needed to give it a try at least.

She'd call him when she got back.

February 1998

She deliberately hadn't made plans for the day itself, in case John popped round to wish her a happy birthday, thinking of perhaps doing a bit of planting if the rain held off, and if she felt up to it. It was grey but mild for the time of year.

She hated birthdays. For some reason they reminded her of being a teenager, waiting for her mum to come back home. And that disappointment, every single time, when her mum's card would arrive, containing nothing but empty wishes for a happy birthday, bracketed by little platitudes that anyone could have said, never once acknowledging her own role in helping to ensure that every birthday since she had left would be an unhappy one.

When it came to it, Olivia did agree to let John out of her sight for a few minutes and Frankie was thrilled when he called in for a coffee at about eleven. She received a little card from Bobbi, too, tucked into a copy of the only P. D. James that Frankie hadn't already read. She was so touched that she picked up the phone to tell her how delighted she was, but there was no-one there.

After John left, she reheated a bowl of tomato soup for lunch but no sooner had she sat down in the garden, than it started raining. So she took the tray into the living room and sat with the book on her knee, and the phone by her side, waiting for the shower to pass. Her face felt heavy and as the tears started to come, she felt suddenly, frighteningly, old.

She rested her feet on the little footstool and thought she'd just close her eyes for a few moments before clearing away the lunch things.

But she must have nodded off.

Because the next thing she knew, the book was at her feet.

She was conscious that she must have heard a noise. But when she looked out of the window there was no-one there.

And yet she felt a very strong presence – as if someone were in the house.

She looked around her. And then she looked back out of the window. There was definitely no-one there, but when she went into the hallway to check, she noticed that the front door was unlocked. She was certain she'd locked it. She checked her keys. They were on the little side table, where they always were.

And so, after locking and firmly bolting it, she headed upstairs just to double-check.

The house was quiet.

And then the phone rang.

It made her jump. She hesitated a beat before going back downstairs to answer it, only to find that it was not on the sofa where she'd left it.

She followed the sound into the kitchen, glancing around the room.

A tiny blue flicker caught her eye.

She gasped, rushed to turn off the hob, checking twice – three times – that everything was switched off.

Her face throbbed and the phone kept ringing.

'Oh, shut up,' she shouted, looking wildly around.

The phone was in the middle of the table – half-hidden under a tea towel.

How could she be so stupid? She threw open the back door and the windows, as the phone rang on and on.

'Oh, what is it?' She picked it up. 'Hello?' she demanded.

She could hear breathing but the person didn't say anything.

'Hello?' she said again. 'Can you hear me?'

The person cleared his throat.

But still he said nothing.

She pulled the receiver away from her ear and held it there, in mid-air, just for a moment, unsure what to do, before slamming it down.

Her ear was hot.

And then a few seconds later it rang again.

She waited until the fifth ring before picking it up carefully, holding it a little distance from her ear before speaking. Her hand was trembling.

'Hello, Frances,' said a voice after a long delay.

'Michael?' She laughed out loud and fell gratefully into a chair. 'Is it really you? How *are* you? Was that you just now? You nearly gave me a heart attack.'

There was a fizzing noise and the voice overlapped with hers.

'I need you to...'

She waited.

'Happy birthday, by the way...'

'Oh, thank you,' she said, distracted by the echo of her own voice. It sounded higher-pitched than the one in her head. 'Did you get my—'

'I need you to—' He stopped.

'What were you going to—' she started.

But there was no reply.

She clenched her teeth. 'Where are you, Michael?' she said, more urgently now. 'What's going on?'

There was a long pause and she heard another voice in a foreign language interfering with the line.

'I'm in Reading,' he said eventually.

'Reading?' Her mouth hung open. 'For God's sake, Michael, where have you been?' She felt panicked. 'What—'

'I'm in trouble. Can you come and get me?' Although he was speaking slowly his voice sounded more distant now and the line was fragmenting.

'What? Now? Well...' She looked all around her and tried to think of something to say. 'Not easily.' She tried to speak louder. 'Can't you get a train?'

'I'm in danger,' he shouted.

She tried to sit up straighter, to steady her breathing. 'Are you alright?'

And then the line went dead.

'Michael? Michael!' she shouted, frantically looking all around her and wondering what on earth she was going to do next.

September 1998

When she got back to her room, she felt pleasantly warm and weary. She thought she'd have a quick shower and a lie down and then head out towards the edge of the town to that walled restaurant that she'd spotted on one of her early morning walks.

Maria, the landlady, was leaning against the gate watering the bougainvillea. Frankie greeted her cheerfully in Greek as she reached for her key. The old woman let out a cry of dismay, clutching Frankie's face and gesturing to the sky. 'This sun.' She pinched Frankie's cheek and tapped the back of her neck as she shook her head.

'I know, I know,' Frankie apologised with a smile. 'I forgot my hat, silly me.'

The old woman didn't say anything more but she stayed where she was, staring at her as she retreated to her room, a look of horror etched on her face.

Frankie was sure it was an overreaction but when she got undressed and went into the bathroom she gasped as she caught her reflection in the mirror. She was fluorescent. Her face in particular was a deep crimson, glistening, like pork crackling. And the skin around her eyes looked swollen. There was a tangle of angry red stripes across her neck and shoulders to indicate where the halter neck of her bikini top had not been. She looked as if she were wearing a white vest.

She raised her hands to her cheeks to try to cool them.

But the heat burnt straight through. And when she turned on the shower the water came out too fast, lashing her across the shoulders like a whip.

February 1998

She tried calling the number back but there was no answer.

After the twentieth time a man picked up. He sounded incoherent and Frankie wasn't sure he had understood what she had said, as she pleaded with him, emphatically, to pass a message to a Michael Webb, to ask him to call his mother.

But Michael did not call.

She tried again, all evening, but no-one picked up.

She lay awake until the early hours of the morning, resolving to catch the very first train to Reading. She knew it was ridiculous. There was no way she would just randomly bump into Michael. But there was no point just sitting around at home either, was there?

She phoned the number again, so tired, now, that she could barely see what numbers she was dialling.

She would call again when she had checked train times.

'I'll call again,' she said to herself as the phone rang and rang, clutching the receiver so tight that her hand ached, unsure whether there was anyone even remotely nearby at the other end who might have somehow magically heard her, let alone understood.

But the next day, when she went downstairs, she found a letter on the doormat addressed to a Mrs Callum Webb.

She recognised the handwriting immediately and checked again that the door was locked.

Dear Frances,

I'm sorry to write with such bad news but you need to know that Michael's back from his trip. He's been back a while, in fact.

He's actually in Bullingdon prison.

She almost dropped the letter. Her vision had gone all blurry and she couldn't absorb the meaning.

Surely this was some kind of joke? Her head ached behind her eyes.

He'd taken one of the vans. He'd been practising for his driving test but he normally asked before using it. I needed it that morning and had no idea where it was. I obviously thought it might have been him – just playing with it – but I had to report it straight-away because of the shotgun in the back. He said he didn't realise it was there and I gave him the benefit of the doubt but what an idiot.

She stopped, confused. The police hadn't mentioned a van, had they? She tried to remember exactly what they'd said as she reread it.

He'd used that phrase before: 'playing with it'.

She felt a strange tingle in her jaw, and as she read on, the paper shook in her hand.

It was shortly before Michael was born.

And she wondered if he had used it again deliberately here – whether he remembered what he'd said that night – or whether it was a coincidence.

I've got it back now, thank God.

They were pretty lenient, given the circumstances. I did my best, as you can imagine. But it's serious. He's been in since November. He didn't want you to know but I felt it was only fair to tell you, especially since he'll be out any day now.

She shook her head in disbelief.

I've said he can stay with me but who knows what he'll do. I wanted to warn you.

It would be good to catch up when all this has blown over.
Callum.

Frankie sat very still, resting her head against the wall as she read and reread the letter until she knew the words by heart.

And after a while her head jerked forwards and she realised that she had nodded off.

Her neck was stiff and she felt so peculiar, almost as if she were jet-lagged, that she stuffed the letter back into the envelope, pressed the seal closed, and dropped it on the mat where she had found it.

And then she went straight back upstairs to bed.

She was woken by the sound of the cordless phone. She jumped. She was still in bed and it was midday. Where was the phone? The newspaper was scattered all over the bed. She looked around her, disoriented, suddenly remembering Michael again and Callum's letter. And the prison.

When she rubbed her eyes, her skin felt greasy and she noticed black ink on the back of her hands. She must have fallen asleep with her arm on the newspaper. She spotted the phone on the floor and reached down.

'Michael?' She dreaded the reply.

'Frances? Can you call me back? I'm—'

She sat up. 'Michael? Is it really you?' She clung to the receiver in case she lost him again.

'I'm in a payphone.'

'Are you really in prison? When did you—'

'I'm out. I got out yesterday. I've got to be quick. Have you got a pen?'

'Yes, of course. Wait a sec...' She scrabbled for her biro. It was tucked inside the newspaper and had already left a thin trail of black on the white duvet cover beneath.

'I've got the number here.'

She smiled deeply, in spite of herself, as she waited for him to go on. 'Where are you, Michael?'

'I'm in Reading.'

'Yes, I know but where in Reading? And *why* are you in Reading, more to the point?' she barked. 'I got a letter from your dad. He said—'

'Someone gave me a lift.' His voice sounded different – deeper – further away. 'Can you come and get me? I'm staying near the fairground just off the main road, near the station.' He spoke very quickly. 'Go to the fairground. Tell them you're looking for Alderton. Number eight. I need some money. Can you bring some of my clothes too? I'm going to get cut off in a minute.'

She felt her chest tighten and she sat up straighter. 'Yes. Don't move from there,' she shouted down the phone. 'I'll come right away.' She looked at her watch. 'I'll be there in an hour or so. I'll just quickly have something to eat first. Where exactly shall I—'

But the line went dead.

'Michael?' she shouted.

She hung up and redialled the number six or seven times, checking obsessively that she had got it right, but nobody answered.

The phone rang while she was finishing her sandwich.

'Michael,' she said, already exasperated as she pulled on her coat. 'I'm just setting off—' She stopped. 'Michael? Are you there?'

She could hear someone. But they said nothing.

In the distance came muffled voices from a television or a radio.

She thought she heard a dog whine. The rhythm of the breathing changed. It sounded closer; she could almost feel the hot breath in her ear.

And then a rustling, like newspaper.

'Who is this?'

The person didn't reply.

'Leave me alone.' She hung up. And stared at the telephone. She'd completely forgotten what she'd been doing.

Her heart was beating too fast and she felt sick.

And then it rang again.

On the third ring she snatched it up. 'Who is this?' she demanded.

'Oh, I'm sorry.' It was a man's voice, loud and deep. 'It's Omar here – Omar Nasr?' She didn't recognise the name. 'From the *Oxford Times?*' He sounded slightly uneasy. 'Is that Phoebe?'

'What?' Her mind went blank.

'I'm sorry, I think I must have the wrong number.' He laughed. 'No worries. I was looking for a Phoebe—'

'Oh, *Phoebe*.' She gripped the phone. 'Did you say Phoebe?' She tried to laugh but it came out like a growl. 'Sorry, I didn't hear you properly. Yes, she's just in the other room. One minute...' She held her hand over the receiver. 'Phoebe, it's for you,' she called out, voice wavering.

She cleared her throat. What on earth had she been thinking? What was she going to say to this man? What had possessed her to call herself Phoebe? How was she going to get round that one?

She counted to ten under her breath and then put the phone to her ear again. 'Hello?'

'Phoebe?' The man sounded as though he was smiling. 'Hi, my name's Omar. From the *Oxford Times?* I got your note.'

'Oh, right. Hi, Omar,' she said, trying hard to sound simultaneously casual, kind, fun-loving and a little bohemian. 'Sorry, did you try and call a few minutes ago?'

'Excuse me?'

'Oh, nothing. Must have been a wrong number.' She couldn't concentrate on what he was saying, distracted by the possibility that it could be Michael, not Callum, making those calls, not to mention the fact that she would have to leave in the next five minutes if she wanted to catch her train to find her son. And so, to hurry things along a bit, she found herself suggesting, to her astonishment, that they just meet up. In Oxford, if that was convenient? Maybe somewhere outside? In a couple of weeks or so?

'Yes,' she agreed. Port Meadow *would* be lovely. 'No, I love boats. I'd love to go out on the boat but maybe we could, you know, start on land? Play it by ear?'

She frowned, picturing her dead body as it floated downstream through the darkness.

'Perhaps, sort of, late afternoon time? Only if you'd like to, though,' she added, stuttering, 'and if the weather's nice enough, obviously.'

She bit her lip, glancing at the clock.

'Maybe a walk?'

The rain was growing heavier and as she got off the train Frankie cursed herself for not bringing an umbrella. The sleeves of her charcoal-grey woollen coat were sodden and she pulled her scarf over her head to fashion a hood, hurrying over the bridge away from the station, dragging the little suitcase behind her.

She could see the pink and green metal machinery and flashing lights of the fairground through the sparsely wooded scrubland. Towering over the treetops stood a gigantic metal grasshopper dressed as a ringmaster. And as she approached, the shivering cedars giving way to a vast concrete car park, the music got louder – deadened dance music without lyrics or dancing.

There was a gust of wind. She looked up. It was as if the wind were physically blowing the rain from the clouds. A line of elm trees cowered, their boughs bending like a congregation at prayer.

Frankie stepped awkwardly over the tarpaulin walkway. The puddles had converged to form a stagnant beige pool and she had to jump to cross it. She looked around. A pregnant woman with a pushchair huddled under the rim of the carousel while a man with wild jack-in-the-box eyes ran in loops to follow his child.

She approached the kiosk. A teenage girl with dyed blonde hair scraped on top of her head and a younger boy in a white tracksuit were playing on a Game Boy. Just behind them was a static caravan with a number plate hanging off – a pile of what appeared to be large black gas canisters dumped at its doorstep. She clutched her handbag more tightly.

'Excuse me,' she said to the girl, who stared back blankly. 'I'm looking for a Michael Webb.'

The girl shrugged and looked back down at the game.

She hesitated. 'He said to ask for Alderton? Number eight, I think?'

The girl pointed across the car park without looking up. 'Over there. Alderton Gardens.'

Frankie was astonished. 'Thank you.' She looked up with a big smile, accidentally catching the eye of a man leaning against the ghost train, smoking a cigarette.

Number eight, Alderton Gardens, was a Victorian terraced house not far from the hospital. A single grey bin with a broken lid lay on its side in the patch of weed-stitched gravel that was the only discernible evidence of anything that might once have resembled a garden. The house next door was pristine, with a pushchair outside – the maroon front door newly painted and the windows catching the early sunlight. But Michael's house was all boarded up – the letterbox was blocked and one of the upstairs windows was missing a pane; someone had taped a patch of cardboard over the bottom left-hand corner.

When she knocked there was no reply.

She peered in the downstairs window. A bearded man in grey tracksuit bottoms and no top was sitting in front of the TV, hunched over a low table, drinking a can of Coke. He looked up but gave no indication of having seen her.

She recoiled and double-checked the door number. It definitely said eight.

She knocked again.

He got up this time and opened the door without saying anything before sitting back down on the sofa.

'Hello,' she said, hesitating before stepping in. 'Is Michael here? Michael Webb?'

He ignored her.

She gave a nervous laugh. 'Michael?' she called.

There was no reply.

'Michael,' she called again, louder this time to make herself heard over the screeching canned laughter from the television. She reached for the doorknob to steady herself.

She heard a movement from upstairs and then someone called down. 'Is that you, Frances?' His voice was scratchy as if he had been asleep.

'Yes.' She glanced at the man before closing the door behind her.

She hovered in the entrance for a moment, not sure where

to look. The floor was covered in rubbish – old magazines, cigarette packets, wrappers and plastic food containers.

She stepped her way through to the kitchen.

The air stank of stale smoke mixed with a curious acrid chemical sort of smell, like clothes that have been put away damp, reminding her, for some reason, of the farm – silage, maybe, or that anti-caking agent stuff Callum used to put in the sheep feed.

She breathed through her mouth.

It was impossible to see the kitchen surfaces through the piles of dirty plates, glasses and takeaway cartons. There were cigarette lighters scattered everywhere, and in the middle of the kitchen stood a plastic laundry basket full of wet clothes. She looked over at the washing machine. It was full.

The walls were bare except for a little chipboard. And on it was pinned a tiny glossy black and white photo that curled at the edges. She looked more carefully and realised it was a scan of a foetus. She grimaced.

And when she turned around Michael was suddenly there, right next to her. 'Oh my God,' she muttered.

He was very thin and pale, dressed in a khaki military over-coat – the epaulettes much too broad – with his hair longer than usual.

'Nice to see you!' she exclaimed, feeling a wave of repulsion. 'Are you off out somewhere?' She tried to force a smile as she swallowed firmly, reaching for the work surface. It was greasy and she snapped her hand away.

'Just cold.' He tried to smile back but it was as if his mouth wasn't working properly, drawing attention to his teeth which were stained.

'Oh, Michael...' She instinctively ran her tongue over her front teeth behind her closed lips.

His right eye was partly closed – the eyelid yellow and puffy.

She felt her face twitch and didn't know what to say. She stumbled towards him and patted him awkwardly on the arm but he withdrew from her. 'How are you?'

'Oh, not so bad.' His lips were dry, cracked with blood.

'I wouldn't have recognised you.' She tried to hold back the tears.

'Yes, you would.' He looked away. 'Have you got the money?'

She gave a reluctant nod. 'What do you need it for?'

'A car,' he said, giving a weird smile, his eyes too pale – pupils like pinpricks.

'Really?' She frowned.

'And some rent.'

'Right. There are a few pairs of jeans – jumpers and stuff here.' She gestured to the suitcase but made no movement to hand it over. 'But I haven't got that much cash, Michael. What are you going to do when it runs out?'

'I doubt I'll need much more,' he said, with a yawn.

'You can't stay here, Michael,' she whispered, gesturing to the work surfaces. 'It's disgusting.'

'None of this matters, Frances. It's what's in here that counts,' he said, tapping his chest. One of his fingernails was missing and she bit her lip.

'Well, what is it exactly you've got in there at the moment?' she snapped. 'It doesn't look as though it's doing you the slightest good. For God's sake, come home with me. I'll make an appointment with Dr Carmichael. You need to get some drops for that eye, for a start. Come on, I'm not taking no for an answer.'

But he wasn't listening. 'How's John?'

'Oh,' she stepped back. 'Yes, he's okay. I don't know if you got his letters – about the wedding and the—'

'Yeah, I did. Tell him he shouldn't marry her, though.'

'Olivia? Why not? What's wrong with her?'

'She doesn't understand what matters,' he said, both eyes closing now, as if he were falling asleep standing up. 'I've got a bad feeling about the wedding.'

'Michael?' She shook him by the shoulders.

'Hello, Frances,' he said eventually, smiling weakly as if surprised to find her still standing there. 'Have you got the money?'

'This picture, Michael.' She pointed to the little scan photograph. 'Whose baby is that? Is the mother here? It's not safe for...' She felt as though she was going to cry. 'This is no place for a baby. Look at all this... this...' She gestured all around her in despair.

He nodded solemnly.

She paused as the enormity of the situation hit her. 'It's not yours, is it, Michael?'

'Mine? My child?' he asked, turning to look at the picture, a strange expression on his face, as if he were seeing it for the first time. He gave her a smile. 'No, of course not.'

'Well, where's its mother?' she hissed, unbuttoning her coat and looking around anxiously for a cloth or some sort of evidence of soap.

But Michael just nodded. Very slowly, his eyes began to close again.

'Oh, for God's sake, Michael!' She grabbed him, shaking him awake. 'Will you please—'

There was a knock at the door. She jumped.

The man in tracksuit bottoms got up to open the door to a thin young man with long shiny dark hair in a ponytail, wearing a navy football shirt and neon red trainers. He was leaning on his bike. Frankie stared at him in terror as she turned back to her son. 'Who are these people?' she whispered.

Michael reached for her arm. 'Can you go now?'

'No. Not until you—'

He closed his eyes again. 'It's just a test,' he muttered.

She grabbed his damp hand and stuffed the wad of notes in his palm, clamping his fingers down to hold it there.

'Thank you,' he muttered.

She didn't look back at him as she marched out of the front door, clutching her handbag.

The man on the bike stepped aside to let her pass, smiling to reveal stumpy brown gums. He winked at her. 'Buenas tardes,' he said, gently rolling away the 'r' of the afternoon.

September 1998

That evening, keen to make the most of her final night on the island, Frankie set out early, as soon as she had finished concealing her sunburnt face under thick layers of face powder, which did the job but gave her a rather ghoulish appearance.

Although she could picture the walled restaurant perfectly – around the corner from an Orthodox church – she couldn't remember exactly where it was. She tried a couple of streets but kept coming back to the main square. In the end she set off down a narrow street that led off from one corner of the square, lined on either side with enlarged black and white photographs of the excavation of Knossos.

At the end of the street, she was pleased to see the church – to one side of a little courtyard, with steps going down to the entrance. An elderly woman, dressed in black with bright white hair beneath a black headscarf, was sitting – a string of prayer beads in her hand – on a broken plastic chair at the top of the steps. She raised a hand to Frankie as she paused to peer inside the church and gestured to her to go inside.

March 1998

As the time drew near for her date with Omar Nasr, Frankie grew increasingly nervous. She was ashamed to face up to the fact that she hadn't been out with anyone else since Callum, not even for a coffee, and she was worried that she wouldn't know how to be.

She'd made a hair appointment for the day before the date. And on her way home, she paused in the window of French Connection, catching sight of her reflection. She turned her face to one side, admiring the way that Nadia, the hairdresser, had taken one look at Frankie's little photograph from twenty years earlier and looked her square-on in the mirror, resting both hands on Frankie's shoulders as she pulled Frankie's hair down, hard, on both sides, to assess the length and reassured her – eyes of steel – that it would be 'easy-fucking-peasy'. She'd do the same shape but make it messier – more modern – so that the fringe, feathered and long, fell in a sweep on one side – 'a bit more sexier – you know – bit more Nicole Appleton'.

A shop assistant had stepped into the window display. She was tall with cropped black hair and long tangerine fingernails, struggling to carry two mannequins dressed only in Sale tee-shirts, one under each arm. She disappeared, returning a few moments later with a fully dressed model, in a red gingham shirt dress, half undone, so that a navy and white striped triangle bikini top was just visible over one plastic shoulder. On its feet was a pair of soft silver leather espadrilles – with wedged rope soles, high enough for Callum to classify as slutty but low enough to go for a walk in without breaking her neck, she reasoned.

With chunky gold ankle straps.

Frankie darted into the shop, grabbed the exact same outfit minus the bikini, and took them to the counter. The assistant smiled at her. 'Such a cool dress,' she said in a bored voice, driving the fabric under a thick white plastic groove in the counter before pliering off the security tag like an electrician cutting a faulty wire. She nodded to the display on the till as she started to fold the clothes, gazing out of the window. 'That'll be £84.99.'

Frankie stared at her, alarmed by the amount, and wondering now if she shouldn't just tell her that she'd changed her mind. She was going to cancel the date and walk straight out.

But instead, she pulled out her cheque book, hand trembling, lulled only by the reassuring sound of the assistant's gold bangles that simmered against the Formica counter like brushed cymbals, her fingernails tapping along in syncopated sympathy as she fed the neat pile into an enormous cardboard bag with rope handles.

The next day at the surgery Debbie kept asking Frankie where she'd had her hair cut – said how it made her look ten years younger and how she should wear it in that style 'forever', speculating, in a stage whisper, with all the regular elderly patients, on whether Frankie had a new man in her life.

Frankie snapped at her in the end, blurting out that she had a date later and she'd appreciate it if Debbie refrained from sharing her ill-informed opinions on her personal life with every Tom, Dick or Harry who happened to be passing their desk to deposit a urine sample.

Because the truth was, although she couldn't wait to get changed into the new outfit, she was so nervous that she could barely speak, let alone eat her packed lunch or interact with any sense of normality with the patients.

The hours passed more slowly than usual and when four o'clock finally arrived she almost shot out the door and raced home to get changed, dismayed when she arrived to see that the main bin in the front garden had fallen over. It was lying on its side with the lid propped against the hedge. She assumed the foxes must have been at them again – trailing rubbish all across her front step: a not-quite-empty can of chopped tomatoes; old newspapers; tea bags and a mush of cooked porridge.

She stared at it all for a moment and then looked around. The street was empty.

She swore under her breath as she stepped over the mess to go inside to get something to sweep it up with.

But when she had finished clearing it all up she was surprised to see a crushed cigarette end on the hallway carpet. She hesitated, mentally calculating the distance from the letterbox. It must have been on the sole of her shoe, she reasoned, lifting her feet to check them. She picked it up, pincered between two fingers, noticing a small grey patch, not quite scorched, but as if it had been trodden on to extinguish it, right there.

She felt faint.

The house was quiet except for the hollow clicking of the kitchen clock.

She darted outside to throw it in the bin before hurrying back in, locking the door firmly behind her.

But when she went into the kitchen to wash her hands, she didn't feel very well. Her head had started to ache and she had a flash of worry, from nowhere, that something had happened to the boys. Her heart was beating too quickly and she wondered, as she sat down with a glass of water, if she should retrieve that cigarette butt to see if she could see the brand, questioning for a moment whether it was such a good idea to go out that evening after all.

She decided against it. It probably wasn't Callum – probably wasn't anyone, in fact. But maybe it would be better to have an early night.

She went upstairs to check everything was okay, hesitating in the doorway to her bedroom. The sash window was open a few inches at the bottom.

She stared at the gap. She didn't even remember opening it in the night. How unlike her to forget to close it. She slid the little brass lock firmly across, relieved to see the bed was just as she'd left it, her new clothes laid out neatly on the duvet cover, shoes still in their box.

She went back downstairs to retrieve the newspaper, turning reluctantly to the TV pages, hesitating briefly to check the crossword was exactly as she had left it that morning.

'Oh, get a grip, Frankie,' she muttered, ripping the page out of the paper and chucking the rest of it aside as she headed back up to get changed.

They had agreed to meet outside a pub on the river, at the edge of the meadow. That way, they could either start walking from there, or go inside if it was raining.

Frankie was a few minutes early so she thought she'd have another go at some of the crossword clues that she hadn't managed to get over breakfast. She retrieved the scrap of ripped-out newspaper from her bag and, rooting around for a biro, she levered herself up to sit on the stone wall, scraping the back of her heel as she did so, wincing as she looked around to check no-one had noticed. She smoothed down the full cotton skirt of the dress, which – underneath her navy and white striped long-sleeved tee-shirt – had made her feel a little bit like Jean Seberg on the Boulevard Saint-Germain earlier, as she strolled down the High Street, checking over her shoulder at one point when she had a feeling that someone was watching her. She now discovered to her annoyance that it had snagged at the back – a large rip just below the knee, somewhat spoiling the effect.

'Phoebe,' came a loud voice.

She jumped and nearly fell backwards off the wall.

'It must be.'

She blushed.

He was tall – very tall, in fact – and large all over – not fat, exactly but thick-set. He had wavy black hair that was untidy and was wearing jeans with a heavy bottle-green jumper with flecks of yellow and blue in the knit, which drew attention to the green of his eyes. Although he was smiling he was staring at her quite intensely and it made her feel shy.

'Hi,' she said, trying to hold his gaze.

'I knew it was you.' He shook her hard by the hand. 'I've been right behind you for about half an hour.'

Alarmed, she looked around to see if there was anyone nearby.

He laughed. 'Sorry. I'll start again. I mean, I happened to be coming the same way as you and I don't know why, but I was convinced it was you.' He gestured to the wall. 'Do you mind if I…?'

'No, please.' She shuffled along, noticing the way he glanced at her ankles as he sat down next to her, his feet flat on the ground – almost concealed by his jeans that were faded and soft – in old-fashioned brown Adidas trainers.

'And then when you turned down Abbey Road and straight towards the meadow…'

His hands were large and expressive and the nails, cut very short, were perfectly rounded.

'I had to hold back a bit and stop myself calling out to you. Because I thought, well, if it's not Phoebe, then I'll be way too close and then still have to walk the rest of the way across the meadow – right behind this beautiful woman – and there's no way that scenario's going to look anything but really weird – if not downright criminal – and it would definitely make the remainder of the journey a *lot* more stressful for everyone involved.' He laughed. 'But it also occurred to me, I guess maybe it might not be her, because she doesn't look at all lonely.' He winked.

'Lonely?' said Frankie, sitting up straighter. 'Who says she's lonely?'

'Why else would someone like that be answering some crappy advert from someone like this?' He pointed two thumbs at himself, those eyes flickering to her mouth.

'Oh, I don't know.' She pretended to appraise him. 'You're not *so* revolting.'

'Thank you.' He laughed. 'I think...'

'And are *you* lonely?' she asked, brushing her hair out of her eye, feeling a confidence that she hadn't felt in years.

'No,' he said carefully. 'I don't know. A little, perhaps.'

'So why did you put an advert in the paper then?'

'Do you really want to know?' He looked at her, suddenly serious. 'Well, I was married.'

She nodded.

'We split up – a few years back – but I haven't really wanted...' He trailed off. 'I wasn't ready to start meeting other people, really.'

She waited for him to go on.

'There's always so much pressure, it seems. Well – in my

family, specifically. In Egypt,' he added, gesturing politely towards the meadow. 'Shall we walk, by the way? Sorry, did I mention… Do you know Egypt?'

'Yes.' She was nodding. 'I mean no.' She concentrated on getting down off the wall. 'I've heard of it, obviously.'

She flushed.

How could she say such an idiotic thing?

Who, in the world, *hadn't* heard of Egypt?

He offered her his hand.

'Thanks. I mean I haven't been there,' she clarified hurriedly.

'Well, you must,' he said simply, setting off towards the river with a long, loping stride. 'There's nowhere like it. But it can be stifling – this expectation that you have to get married – hundreds of children – just follow this path that everyone expects you to follow. I knew I didn't want that. I wanted to take my time – have some fun first. It's part of the reason I moved here, I guess, for art college. Had no idea I'd end up staying all these years.'

There was a luminosity to his eyes that reminded her of someone. He looked as though he wanted to say something else but he stopped himself and looked the other way instead at a clump of willows leaning over the water. 'What about you?'

'Pretty similar, I guess,' she said. 'In some ways. Not the Egypt bit, obviously.'

Why did she say that?

Why was she being so weird?

'I'm separated, too, I mean. And haven't really felt like dating much, either.'

Until about fifteen minutes ago, she decided.

He nodded but seemed preoccupied.

'Actually, that was a lie,' he said.

Frankie glanced warily at him.

'I might as well get it out the way early on.'

He stared at her for too long, as if he wasn't sure whether to say something.

And then he took a deep breath. 'My daughter died.'

'Oh.' Frankie stopped. Her hand rushed to her mouth. 'I'm so sorry. That's—'

'Thanks, no. It's okay,' he said awkwardly, staring at the ground. 'Shall we…?' He hesitated before carrying on walking.

Some teenagers were sitting on the back of a houseboat, fishing. They watched them approach.

'I mean, it's not okay… obviously. She was hit by a car. It'll be eight years in November. Crossing the road – with her mum – in Headington; the guy driving just didn't see her. She was only three.'

'Oh, that's too awful.' She didn't know where to look. 'That's just—'

'It is, isn't it?' He stared right at her, frowning in concentration.

They walked in silence for a while. And when he spoke again he didn't look at her but stared straight ahead at the boats passing as if he were back at the scene of the accident, watching the cars stream past but frozen to the spot.

'She just wriggled away from Lorna – from her mum. Blink of an eye. He didn't see her,' he said again. 'She couldn't… nobody could *do* anything.' He shook his head. 'I was at home. They just popped out to the park. Funny thing was that I'd had half a mind on going with them that day. It was nothing special. But then for some reason I just didn't.' He stopped, silent for a while.

'I'm so sorry,' Frankie said. 'I don't know what to say.'

'Thank you.' He turned to her. 'I blamed my wife. I couldn't forgive her. I'm so ashamed now. But I couldn't even look at her. There was nothing she could have done. I knew that, on an intellectual level. But honestly? I *hated* her for letting it happen – letting go of her hand – taking that most precious life away from me.'

'Right.' Frankie nodded. Her face stung.

'I couldn't bear it. I thought it was going to suffocate me.' He looked right at her and then he suddenly seemed to come to his senses. 'I'm sorry. Why am I telling you all this? This is way too intense.' He gave a hollow laugh. 'Okay, so now you can see why I find it quite hard to meet people—'

'No – please. Go on.' She spotted a patch of stone on the riverbank like a miniature jetty. 'Shall we sit down, by the way?'

'Good idea.' He took off his shoes and rolled his jeans up over his ankles before swinging his feet down into the water. She sat down next to him.

'She couldn't forgive herself either. Who would? And we tried for a couple of years. But we couldn't make it work – couldn't get beyond it. There was just this big hole – like a heavy imprint,' he said, pressing his hands together, 'in the middle of our little family, where, having been three, suddenly – one day, just like that – we were back to being two again. One life neatly subtracted. But with the two of us impossibly changed. Reduced – forever – by Reem not being there.'

She nodded. An image of Michael as a baby flashed through her head.

She looked down at the water, her jaw heavy.

'I couldn't stop thinking about all the lives she'd never touch, the people she'd never know or love. It seemed like such a spectacular waste. And I had no-one here – except Lorna, obviously. And I'd never appreciated how lonely this place can be.' He gestured to the wide expanse of meadow. 'People were suddenly so closed. Tucked away in their houses with the blinds down and the gates shut. I couldn't stand it. I'd noticed it before, subconsciously, but when Reem died I hit a wall.'

He shook his head and looked into the distance.

'It must have been unbearable.'

'Yeah. Do you know what the worst bit was?' He turned to her. '*No-one* mentioned it. They either avoided us. Or just talked around it – about things that don't matter enough to upset anyone. I hated it. Missed Egypt almost as much as I missed Reem, somehow – got them mixed up somewhere in my heart.'

He breathed out deeply.

'I understood, then, what it all means – what comes of having all these people looking out for each other – sticking their noses in each other's lives.' He paused.

'Being there,' she said.

He nodded.

'I thought about going back, when Lorna and I split. But I found I couldn't leave this place. Because this was where Reem was. Stuck in this horrible in-between land in my own head. Despair, I suppose you'd call it. For a long time.'

They were quiet for a while. 'So how did you start to come through it?' she said tentatively.

'Well, I'd built up a bit of a community at the university. And it struck me, after a while, that if I didn't find a way to keep living – if I carried on, alone, just immersed in my grief like that – then I might leave nothing behind, either. Like a ghost.'

He stopped.

'Okay. Permission to leave.' He tried to laugh but when he looked over at her she caught a glimmer of fear in his eyes.

'Oh, don't be silly.' She rested a hand on his arm. 'It's okay.'

'One thing you're going to learn about me is that I never stop talking. I even talk when I'm asleep.'

She didn't laugh along. 'It must have been so difficult to get back up – keep going – after all that.'

He nodded, slowly and firmly, and said nothing – just holding her gaze, steady and calm, so that she no longer felt nervous – quite the reverse, in fact.

Her shoulders fell and she could feel the tension draining out of her, finding herself breathing deeper, sitting straighter, like a plant that someone was pulling gently on a string – guiding her to grow completely and entirely towards the light – not only seen and understood but warmed.

'You're lovely, aren't you, Phoebe?' he said.

Frankie blushed and smiled awkwardly. 'Thank you,' she said, wishing – more than anything – that she hadn't told him her name was Phoebe.

'Anyway, now you've heard my entire life story barely before we've even introduced ourselves; sorry about that, by the way; I'd completely forgotten what I was talking about. As I was saying, turns out after all that I was right.' He laughed. 'It *was* you! And that's another thing you're going to learn about me…' He elbowed her casually in the ribs and whispered, hot in her ear, so that she wobbled and had to reach out for balance, clinging to a clump of grass. 'I'm always right.'

She felt slightly giddy and was concentrating so hard on not blushing that although she was trying to look him in the eye, his gaze – at once so still, so true and so beautiful – unmoored her, as though she would have to look away – nodding and smiling, all the while – to physically prevent herself from falling – not only into the river but also, headlong, into immediate, unpremeditated outdoor acts of love with this devastatingly attractive artist, sitting firmly – alongside her – on very much the right side of forty-three.

September 1998

It was dark inside the church, the air warm, and thick with incense. From every wall hung tapestries, paintings and ikons. An enormous chandelier hung from a domed roof and a handful of people knelt, alone, at pews.

Frankie hesitated before sitting down in the back row. She glanced around to check no-one was watching and then she shuffled along so she could sit, concealed, in the corner.

She closed her eyes, breathing deeply and calmly as she inhaled the pungent incense, her heart steady and strong. It had only been a few weeks since the fire and yet it felt like another lifetime. Since she'd arrived in Greece, she'd felt all the anger seeping gradually out of her, leaving her with an unfamiliar sense of calm that she didn't recognise.

She heard footsteps and checked over her shoulder. An elderly man was lighting a candle, while a child danced in the doorway, silhouetted against the evening sun.

March 1998

The morning after her date with Omar she came downstairs to find a thick letter on the doormat – a padded A4 envelope with no stamp or postmark, addressed simply to a Mrs Callum Webb.

It was definitely Callum's writing. Surely he hadn't got the divorce papers together that quickly? She barely dared to believe it. No, it wasn't possible.

But what else could it be?

And why had he sent it to this address? She frowned as she ripped it open, disturbing a cloud of shredded paper. She must have told them a hundred times to make sure he addressed everything to the solicitor.

It was dated the previous day, which meant he must have delivered it that morning because it definitely hadn't been there when she got home the night before. Her stomach churned. She checked the door was locked.

A little photograph fell out. She picked it up. It was of her, on her honeymoon, on a boat. She was dressed in shorts and a shirt loosely buttoned up over her bikini. Her hair was blowing all over the place and she was tanned and laughing.

Frankie couldn't stop looking at it and felt a deep wrench inside her as she wondered where that person had gone.

Dear Frances,

I've been thinking of you lately.

I've been clearing out the house and came across some old pictures.

Her eyes flickered back to the photograph.

I can still see you, that night in the taverna on the hillside. Do you remember the music? I couldn't take my eyes off you. Nobody could. I didn't want the evening to end. We drank too much but you didn't care.

She stopped, surprised to suddenly remember it all again so vividly, and smiled rather cautiously as she rolled her eyes.

It had been so hot that day. I can still taste the salt on your skin when I finally got you back to the room.

She sat down on the stairs.

I remember thinking that if I died right there, in that very moment, with your smile in my eyes and your body in my arms, no heaven could match that.

Frankie looked up, her mind a blank.

She closed her eyes. Her jaw and shoulders felt heavy.

You were wearing that dress – the green one. Do you remember it? I don't think I ever saw you in it again. I thought I must be dreaming. I couldn't believe how this incredible girl had agreed to be my wife. I kept thinking someone was going to turn up and whisk you away and tell me it was all a big mistake.

I didn't ever want to leave.

Her face stung as she reread the words, the images coming back in a rush, as if there had been no lull. 'Oh, grow up, Frankie,' she muttered.

I want you to know, that after all we've been through, there's not a single day that goes by where I don't think to myself that I'd give up my whole life – the farm – the kids – the lot – to go back to that night – just for a night.

She sighed deeply, her breath coming out in a strange juddering sound.

You were never cut out for a farm. Everyone said so. You were too good for that. Too good for me, I mean. I always knew it was only a matter of time before you realised it too.

I think I must have known all along, even then – even when you swore the opposite – that you'd leave me one day and I'd wind up doing it on my own.

She forced her eyes open too wide, to let the cold air dry up the feelings that were creeping up inside her.

I'm just sorry I waited so long to tell you all this – wasted all those years – but I guess there comes a time in a person's life when there's no need to hide anymore. When the worst has already happened and there's nothing left to fear.

Her breathing quickened but she was struggling to get enough air inside her, as if something were tightening around her throat.

I'm sure Mike's told you about the cows and what a mess they've left us with. There's no way we'll ever get them back. You've heard what they're saying. Even if they don't ban it wholesale; no-one's touching the stuff anytime soon. The sheep are next. I've argued until I'm blue in the face. But they've said there are no exceptions – not if there's been a case.

From nowhere she had a memory; they were feeding the lambs together – how the strength of their jaws always astonished her. The lamb had wrenched the bottle clean out of her hand so that she shot backwards, landing on her backside, covering both of them, head to toe, in milk, while the lamb stared, deadpan, gurning ferociously on the empty teat.

We're bleeding cash, obviously. I've tried everything but there's no way we can bring it back from here – not in such a short time with no-one to hand down to.

Frankie frowned.

Made me realise we could have made that change you always wanted, and kept the dairy on. It's too late now – it's plummeted in value with the rest of it. Might as well sell off the cottage and the back barns, too, while they're still worth anything.

She reread the words carefully to check she hadn't missed anything.

I know it's stupid to even hope. But I can't go to my grave without asking.

All I want is one last chance with you.

Where we can forget about everything that happened.

Can you find it in your heart to think about it?

Callum

Beneath his name he had scribbled the phone number. It was strange seeing it again, so immediately familiar even after all those years.

P.S. Please pass my best regards to John for his big day and tell him that I hope he makes a better job of it all than his old man ever did...

She sat there, staring at the photograph and rereading the letter for the best part of an hour, before heading into the kitchen to find a pen and paper.

And then, before she could do something she knew she would regret for the rest of her life, she sat down at the kitchen table and wrote back to him.

Dear Callum,

She sat, thinking, writing, crossing out, rewriting, allowing herself to go to places she'd never been before – say those things she'd carried inside all those years but had never been able to articulate.

Thank you for your letter.

She wouldn't send it, she decided, on balance, but for once she would have her say.

I must admit it took me by surprise.

Of course I remember that evening. But it was a long time ago, wasn't it? So much has changed since then. I don't feel the same as that girl in the photograph. I feel like a very different person altogether, in fact, but it doesn't make me nostalgic. If anything, it's made me realise how much we've all moved on.

She paused, clamping the pen between her teeth, picturing his face. She crossed out the last sentence before hurriedly adding '*I always will*' after the bit about remembering the evening.

She stared at the page for several minutes without writing anything.

And then something seemed to grip her from the inside. Her jaw was tight and she realised, as she wrote on and on, that she was holding the pen so tightly that her whole forearm was aching.

But she didn't stop.

I haven't loved you for a long time. I loved you once. But I was very young, very naive and very kind. More than that – I was far too forgiving. And you know it.

The trouble is that through all that time, you never once thanked me. And you never, ever, she added, underlining it, *said sorry.*

I was a shell of a person when I left you. You'd worn me down to the bone.

And it took me a long, long, time to build myself back up.

I don't care as much as I used to because I've grown up now and you don't scare me anymore.

The pen jerked as if someone had knocked it out of her hand and she realised her whole body was shaking.

I am very sorry that you are going through such a dreadful situation with the farm. It must be heartbreaking. And I wish you the very best of luck with it all over the coming months. I am sorry I can't help you anymore.

She reread the sentence and crossed out the apology, too hard, so that she tore a little hole in the paper where she had just meant to put a full stop.

But I don't want you to contact me again. Or the boys. And I also noticed that you didn't mention the divorce instructions that Southeys have served.

She reached for the letter from the solicitors to check their wording.

I'm confident that you will act with integrity and deliver the papers by the date – and to the address – requested (supplied again, below, for your information) so we can put the past behind us and move on, once and for all.

Yours,
Frankie.

It took her all morning.

She hadn't even had a cup of tea.

But when she sealed that envelope, she knew that something deep inside her was resolved.

And taking out a fresh sheet of paper Frankie decided to reply to another letter that had arrived almost twenty-five years earlier – from her mother.

Thanks for the little card you sent me on my wedding day. It upset me so much, back then, but I can see now, all these years later, how hard it must have been to say anything at all.

I don't even know if this is still the right address for you or what you are doing these days. But I wanted to let you know that my eldest son, John, is getting married in December. So I thought I'd drop you a note to say you'd be very welcome if you decided you'd like to pop by. No need to reply or anything but I enclose an invitation, just in case.

Love,
Frances.

And then she got dressed, her heart thumping in her chest, and before she could change her mind, she walked to the end of the road, and posted them.

September 1998

Frankie wondered whether she ought to light a candle or say some kind of prayer or something. It had been so long since she'd set foot in a church, she'd forgotten what she was supposed to do. Yes, she'd light a candle, she decided. She'd just wait until those people had gone. She felt silly saying a prayer. She never knew what to say, even though she knew it didn't really matter because no-one could hear her.

Perhaps she would just say a little prayer that the flight home would be safe.

But that felt a bit selfish so she prayed that John and Michael were alright, too.

She breathed deeply, dimly aware of someone walking around behind her. She glanced over one shoulder. A priest in a black hat and long white beard was walking, head down, towards the sanctuary.

And then the noise faded once more to silence.

Her mind went blank. And she felt her mouth pulling downwards as a pressure started to build behind her eyes.

She let them close, breathing in the hot, perfumed smoke.

It took her straight back to the time of the fire.

April 1998

When he had said goodbye, Omar had casually mentioned going for dinner one evening, if she fancied it. And he had called Frankie a couple of days later to ask if she might like to try out a new Lebanese restaurant that he'd spotted on Little Clarendon Street that was just about to open. They ended up chatting for almost an hour before setting a date for a Thursday evening in the middle of April.

And not long after she got off the phone, Frankie had had another call – from Michael. Her ear was still warm.

'I've been trying to get through for ages,' he said.

She raised her eyebrows. 'I was talking to a friend.'

There was something he wanted to ask her, offering to come to *her*, this time. But she thought it would be easier to meet somewhere in between instead, agreeing in the end to his suggestion of a coffee shop in town called Vittorio's, explaining firmly that she wouldn't be available until the weekend unfortunately. But perhaps they could meet first thing on Saturday?

She'd been hoping to make some headway on that decorating, over the weekend, that she'd been resolutely putting off since Michael had left home. It had crossed her mind that if the second date went as well as the first, she might like to invite Omar back to the house afterwards, provided that wouldn't appear too forward.

For although she had come clean, in the end, about her real name and had spoken very briefly about John and Michael, she certainly hadn't told him where she lived yet. She wanted to take things slowly. Well, she reasoned, blushing to recall the way they had parted at the end of their first date, brushing themselves down as they emerged, sheepish and shivering in the moonlight, her new dress ripped before the date had even begun and now almost ruined beyond repair by the long meadow grass; *relatively* slowly, at least. Omar had still been smiling from her awkward confession to having lied about her name: 'I *knew* that was you on the phone… "I'll just go and get Phoebe…"'

And there was nothing so wrong about wanting the house to look nice, was there?

On the Saturday morning, she set off early in case she couldn't find the café Michael had suggested. She hadn't recognised the name Vittorio's and just couldn't picture it when he described the 'little family-run place, round the back of the precinct, behind the betting shop, where you can still get a cup of coffee and an egg roll for £1.95'.

When she got there, she realised she'd been past it hundreds of times but had never noticed the name and certainly never considered actually going inside. Besides, it always looked to be closing down.

The maroon canopy was ripped and the gold italic lettering faded. The windows could do with a good wash, too, she observed with a frown, peering in surreptitiously. But although there was no sign of Michael, there were a couple of people inside. And there was an old-fashioned bell that chimed when she pushed open the door.

The air was hot and greasy under stark orange striplights and the smell of frying meat clung immediately to her clothes.

She thought privately how much better she could run a place like this herself – open a couple of windows for a start, she observed, looking over crossly at an elderly woman on crutches who was leaning – a cushion under one arm – against a Lavazza coffee sign at the counter, chatting to the waitress – a short, bosomy girl with a bored expression who was staring at her reflection in the door of the microwave as she arranged her long pastry-coloured hair into an elaborate twist, like a cinnamon swirl.

Frankie took a seat at the grubby white plastic table in the furthest corner from the counter but kept her coat on. She tried to push her chair out a bit – her face already starting to feel too hot – before realising that the chairs were fixed to the floor.

She heard a sputtering. Across the road, a rusty white Transit van pulled up and parked outside the betting shop. A tall thin boy in a long khaki overcoat got out. It was Michael, she realised abstractedly, her eye drawn back to the van as she watched him cross the road. It was exactly the same sort that Callum used to drive and Frankie felt a funny metallic taste in her mouth.

'Hello, Frances.'

Frankie tried to stand up but there wasn't quite enough space and she found herself squashed awkwardly against the table.

She was startled by how different Michael looked up close – so much so that she wasn't sure at first whether to embrace him or shake him by the hand. Underneath his coat, which was unbuttoned and flapped when he moved, he was wearing a thin black jumper and black drainpipe cords with rather Dickensian lace-up boots and with very short hair, which made him look somewhere between a rock star and a vagrant but undeniably striking and unexpectedly handsome. She noticed the waitress staring at him.

His posture was changed, for a start. He was standing much straighter than the last time she'd seen him, which gave him the air of having grown, considerably. He was clean-shaven, too, and the way his hair was cropped made his face look much more angular than before and his skin – usually so pale – was much clearer, she realised with a sigh of relief, than the last time she'd seen him, and lightly tanned, making the whites of his eyes all the brighter. She was briefly taken aback by how much he resembled Callum at that age. But without that smile.

'Right, shall we get a cup of coffee or something? You look well, Michael.' She was unnerved to feel a strange pang inside. Was it envy perhaps of Michael's youth? Or regret? She quickly pushed the feelings aside. 'So, this must be the car, then?' she said, nodding to the window.

He glanced over his shoulder. 'Thanks for your help with that. Dad was going to get rid of it. It's pretty ancient – but it goes, sort of.'

'Yes, I remember it. I'm astonished he's still got it.' She tried to laugh but a horrible memory flashed vividly through her mind. She could still hear the music that had been playing in the van – too loud – to block out Michael's screams. 'I always hated it, actually.' She coughed and looked around for the waitress. 'You haven't passed your test, though, have you?'

'Of course I have.' He laughed. 'I've been quite busy actually. I've got a job too, you'll be pleased to hear. With Monira. I've been staying with her a couple of weeks.' He paused, watching her reaction. 'But I obviously need to find somewhere a bit more permanent.'

Frankie nodded, her face tight. 'Right,' she said eventually.

'She got that funding that she went for before – from the council. Do you remember? Ages ago? For another post.'

'Great. Congratulations,' she added stiffly.

When the waitress came over to take their order, Frankie was unnerved by the way Michael stared at her, not even looking away when she returned to the counter, and again that expression flashed uninvited through her mind: 'sexually motivated'. She shuddered, strangely tongue-tied.

'I need somewhere to stay, Frances. I think it would be good if I came home with you for a few nights. I am a bit worried about Dad.'

'No way.' She recoiled, sipping her coffee. It was foamy and lukewarm.

His face hardened. 'You've got the space. Don't you think you have a duty, kind of, to share—'

'Absolutely not.' She couldn't think of the right words.

'Well, in that case, what about you help me a bit with some rent? Just until—'

'Until what? Last time I saw you, you could barely speak.' She glanced at her watch and drained her coffee. 'Where did all that money go? What makes you think I've got anything left?' Her eyes narrowed.

Michael looked down at the table. 'Well, that's why I suggested staying with you. It doesn't cost anything that way. And then you won't be on your own.'

'Well, who says I don't *want* to be on my own for a bit?' She stood up. 'Look, I need time to think about this. It's all a bit out of the blue, if I'm honest.'

'Hey, calm down.' He glanced over his shoulder. 'I know it's asking a lot. But if there's anything you can give – anything – it would be a massive help. I promise I'll pay you back. Or if you change your mind and let me come back home for a bit, I can help—'

'No.' She grimaced. 'Well, look, I haven't got much. It's

been an expensive couple of months, as it happens.' She thought about those clothes she'd bought and felt guilty all over again. 'I've got a twenty-pound note.' She rummaged in her handbag and counted out some change. 'And here's three – four pounds – for the coffees and your egg sandwich thing. That should more than cover it.' She flung it down on the table a little too hard.

He didn't move. 'Thank you,' he said eventually, still refusing to look her in the eye. 'I knew you'd help.'

'I'm sorry to dash off.' She lingered. 'Good luck.'

'It's not me who needs luck,' he said, without looking at her. 'Thanks again, by the way, but I do think you're making a mistake.'

She felt all her muscles stiffen and felt an urge to shake him by the shoulders.

She clamped her lips together and took a deep breath.

'Goodbye, Michael.' She kissed him on the cheek and walked away.

And although she wanted to, more than anything, she didn't once look back.

***

Even after all that time the house still felt so quiet with both the boys gone. As she looked around Michael's room, in spite of everything that had happened, she still hated to see all his things tidied away – his books, all neatly stacked – the bed bare. She crossed her arms. It was as if the old Michael – *her* Michael – had died.

By the end of the day, she had cleared out both of the boys' rooms but hadn't even started on the painting. Boxes towered, with menace, above the banisters on the upstairs landing and she resolved to dump the lot of them in the

The Broken Line

shed in the morning and take everything that didn't fit to the charity shop.

The sun had come out unexpectedly that afternoon and the day had grown surprisingly warm. When she finally went up to bed, her bedroom smelt stuffy – like damp towels – and when she opened the sash window, flakes of white paint came off on the heels of her hands. Her muscles ached from lifting and she had barely opened her book before she fell into a sudden, uncompromising sleep.

She cleaned and painted solidly for the whole of the following day. The phone didn't ring. The hours passed too quickly. And she was astonished to find that it was at least four o'clock in the afternoon before she realised she had forgotten to eat lunch. She ached all over and yet felt a deep sense of peace when she finally sat down at the end of the day to watch TV with a glass of wine and some cheese and crackers before collapsing gratefully into bed.

She could only have been asleep for an hour or so when a loud noise woke her. She sat straight up – her pyjamas drenched in sweat – heart racing. She thought she'd heard a thud downstairs; she was sure of it.

She concentrated. She couldn't be certain that she hadn't dreamt it.

Everything was too silent.

And then she smelt something strange – fumes, from the paint, perhaps? It was getting stronger, as she realised, too slowly, how warm the room had grown and how the smell, as it wafted closer, was mixed with something else.

Smoke.

Her mind and her body were momentarily paralysed.

There was a great crash outside the room. It must have been

the bookcase falling, she realised, leaping up, her mouth dry. She looked wildly all around her. She must have left the phone downstairs.

'Fire,' she said aloud, stuttering as the reality of the situation struck her. She reached for the door handle.

It burnt.

She jumped with a yelp, her hand flying to her mouth. The skin throbbed and started to blister almost in front of her eyes.

She could hear a gushing sound outside now – like seawater crashing against the harbour walls.

The house is on fire, she thought, unable to register what was happening.

She whimpered but didn't move.

How was she going to phone? And where was her handbag? She rocked on her feet, unsure what to do.

The window was still open.

She would have to climb out.

She was weeping so much now that everything was blurry. She rushed to the window, calculating her fall. She pushed up the window with all her strength and climbed out on to the window ledge, the splintery wood scraping against her spine.

The street was silent – the houses in darkness. In the distance she saw a dog sniffing the base of the streetlamp. And then a shape – a man, was it? – at the crossroads, almost concealed by the trunk of the plane tree. She felt a surge of hope and called out to him. 'Excuse me.'

But the shape didn't move. Maybe he hadn't heard her. Or maybe there was no-one there.

She craned her head, shouting louder. 'Hello! Can you help, please?' She felt ridiculous. Perhaps she should just jump. It wasn't so far down, was it? She felt a sudden pain in the back of her neck and in her shoulders.

As the sound of the flames grew louder, she clung more desperately to the windowsill, placing her feet further apart to carry her weight more safely as she squatted and carefully lifted her other arm to wave above her head.

But the shape still did not move.

She started screaming, 'Fire!' Surely someone would hear her.

She looked around wildly. It was too dark.

She was going to die. A strange animal noise came out of her and she wiped her eyes with the back of her hand.

'Somebody – please,' she groaned, the heat behind her almost unbearable now. She shouted again, as loud as she could, and waved both arms above her head – her voice so loud that it sounded as if it belonged to someone else. She was almost hoarse.

And then, to her amazement, the man stepped right out from behind the tree, towards the streetlamp, casting a long shadow in the edge of the light so that he looked impossibly tall and thin. 'Hello!' he shouted.

It sounded like Michael.

'Oh, thank God,' she gasped, feeling all the tension in her body fall, like a juddering weight from her shoulders. 'Michael?' she screamed. 'Is that you? The house is on fire.'

She was crying so hard that she could barely see at all. But it didn't matter anymore for she was saved.

But he didn't move. It couldn't have been Michael. Instead, he simply stuck one arm out.

She felt her insides drop.

And then he waved back.

Her vision was failing altogether now and she grabbed hold of the ledge. She realised she had no idea what she could possibly do next.

And then, in an instant, something inside her changed.

She lost all sense of fear. She opened her mouth and shrieked as loudly as she could. 'Help me, you fucker. I'm on fire.' Her throat burnt.

But the man stayed exactly where he was.

She tried to steady her breathing but the room behind her was filling with smoke. It was in her mouth now. She coughed but couldn't get rid of it.

There was no alternative. She was going to have to jump out of the window. She looked down, her body swaying. There was a patch of grass below but it was slightly to the left of the window, and anyway, it was much too far to drop. How would she survive the fall?

She would very likely break her neck, she thought, with a dawning realisation of her own mortality, picturing her broken body, just a heap of bones in the darkness – dumped by the dustbins, for the flies. She cried out like a child.

She could feel the heat of the fire in the walls of the house. And then something crunched. It sounded like part of the roof. She didn't dare look up. A burning ember stung her cheek. She gasped, squashing her face against her shoulder – light-headed now – and her mouth tasted odd, like aniseed.

And then the man whistled and started to walk away.

And at that precise moment she saw something that almost made her heart stop. It was the way the dog stopped completely still before falling immediately into line alongside him.

She stared.

And as the man walked off, there was a sloping stride to his gait that reminded her of Callum.

She shook her head so hard that the man and the dog blurred together.

Callum was bigger – broader.

That man was much too thin, wasn't he?

She tried to regulate her breathing. She forgot all about the jump. Her hands were sweating and she felt she might lose her grip. Her vision was completely grainy now and she knew that she was going to be sick. She looked down. The windowsill was streaked with blood from where her toenail had torn off. She was convulsing.

It wasn't him, she assured herself, over and over, afraid she was losing her mind as the syllables started to blend into each other and the words lost all meaning as the man and the dog were absorbed by the darkness.

But it was the decision that it couldn't have been Callum that made her mind freeze.

Because if it wasn't him, she realised – letting her body fall, finally, to its fate – there was only one other person it could possibly have been.

September 1998

All was dark.

And she felt entirely alone and unseen.

She sat there for several minutes, listening to her breath – quiet and steady – in the warm air.

And without knowing why, she thought she sensed Michael. It was as if he were sitting alongside her. She wondered what he would say. She could almost hear his voice. And she remembered what he always used to say to her. He will forgive you.

She wiped away a tear.

'I'm sorry,' she whispered. 'I'm sorry I pushed you away – that I couldn't be the person you needed me to be. I was just me all along.'

After a while she felt the weight gradually easing from her shoulders and she sat back on the hard pew. 'I didn't do a very good job of it all, did I? What a mess.'

Behind her eyelids she thought she saw him – his face distorting, fragmenting, all at once, into tiny overlapping images – as a baby, a child and a man – all rolled into one.

'What I did was wrong. I'm sorry for not loving you.'

And she thought about it all – the time when Michael was born, finding that her mind replayed it without a gap, as if it had been stored up all along, merely waiting for her – until she was ready.

April 1998

'Your son found you,' the paramedic explained, leaning too close to her face when Frankie awoke, in the ambulance, what felt like days later.

She couldn't feel anything or move her legs.

And she was breathing – ragged and fast – through a mask.

'He was distraught when we arrived – ever so upset, he was. It must have been a dreadful shock for him.'

As she lay there, she closed her eyes.

And for the first time since Michael was a baby she prayed.

She prayed with a faith that she had never felt before, feeling a hot warmth seeping from the place where her deadened legs had once lain up to what must have been her neck. She involuntarily brought up image after image that captured all the fragments and scenes of Michael's life – like untouched frames hanging, hallowed, in a gallery.

Because everything came back to the beginning – the very start of him – an act of vengeance, hate and punishment. There had been no hope for either of them. Who had she been kidding all these years? She was to blame for all the evil he had wrought. She should never have let him be.

And as she lay there, in death's antechamber, she repented with her whole soul, imploring a God that she knew now for the first time. And she prayed that whether she lived or died she would never have to see her son again.

*

Somewhere in the distance a child was singing.

'*The wife wants a child.*'

'*Frankie,*' came a voice.

She felt as though she was on the bottom of the ocean.

'*Ee-ay-ah-di-open your eyes.*'

The nurse was leaning right over her. And she immediately remembered the fire, triggering the images of Michael that dutifully began to race through her head again as if there had been no pause.

'Who was that singing?'

'I'm sorry to wake you, love,' said the nurse, tugging at Frankie's pillow, 'but could you lift your head a fraction?'

'Do you have to do this right now? Couldn't you do it later?' Frankie snapped, her neck straining as she tried to keep her head held up as the pillow was wrenched from beneath her.

'Didn't Tania mention your son's here?'

'Which one?'

'I don't know. He's in reception. Tania, bless her, didn't think to ask his name,' the nurse said loudly, her greasy face reddening as she stuffed the pillow into the clean pillowcase. 'Said something about taking you out to the garden centre.'

'The garden centre?' Frankie's breathing quickened. 'There must be some mistake. Look at me! I can't go to a garden centre. She must have misheard.'

The nurse clicked her fingers twice in front of Frankie's eyes so that she felt her head lurch backwards. 'You're alright, love. It's just the morphine. It's okay, there's no garden centre, more's the pity,' she added with a chuckle. 'That would brighten things up around here, wouldn't it?' Her hair was hanging too close to Frankie's face. It smelt of stale cigarettes. Frankie held her breath as she took too long to plump the pillow beneath her head.

'It's nice to have visitors once in a while, isn't it, Mrs Webb? Let me go and ask his name.'

The stiff white cotton felt pleasantly cold to Frankie's tired cheek and she closed her eyes again, lulled by the whispered ministrations of the nurses in the cubicle opposite.

'Mum.'

She opened her eyes. A man was sitting beside the bed.

He took her hand in his.

'Michael,' she gasped, her thin knuckles white against the flat arms of the bed as she tried to move, forgetting her leg was paralysed. Her eyes darted towards the door. 'Help,' she called out – her breathing hoarse and irregular. 'It's him!'

'Mum, it's me – John.' He squeezed her hand to reassure her.

She screamed.

'It's alright, Mum.' He looked all around and reached over her to press the buzzer.

'Get away from me!' she hollered; her mouth was too dry. 'It's Michael.'

'It's the morphine, Mum. They said it would make you woozy. I've just come to check how you're—'

She opened her mouth to scream again but all that came out was a high-pitched rasping sound like the shriek of a barn owl. A woman came hurrying in, wiping her wet hands on her apron.

'Is everything alright, Frankie?' she said too loudly, in a sing-song voice, glancing warily at John through a strained smile.

'I think she's hallucinating,' he said.

'Get him out of here!' Frankie screamed. 'Don't listen to him. He's dangerous.'

John stood up. 'I'm sorry,' he said. 'I didn't mean to upset her. I was just popping by to see how she was feeling.'

Frankie let out a piercing scream. 'He's trying to kill me!' she shouted. 'It's Michael. Get him away!' She was shaking now and the bed was rocking. The woman reached out a hand to steady it.

'There, there, Frankie, love. No-one's trying to kill anyone. The young man says his name is John. There's no Michael here. He's just come to say hello.'

'Get him away from me!'

An elderly man peered around the door, forehead creased in concern. 'Are you alright?' he checked, as the nurse gently steered him away.

'No!' she shouted. 'Help me! Take them away!' She was crying now – panicked, like a little child, her face trembling.

John picked up his jacket. 'I'll come back in the morning,' he called across to the nurse.

Frankie was finding it hard to breathe properly, the air jerking in and out in rapid, short breaths; one of her eyelids was flickering uncontrollably.

She caught snippets of their conversation as they walked back down the corridor. 'She's had a terrible shock… a bit confused… lucky not to have been very badly burnt.'

She tried to calm her breathing and ignore the bleeping that was coming from the cubicle beside hers while she tried to block out the lines of the song going round and round in her head like a carousel. *Ee-ay-ah-di-oh the child wants a dog…*

'Oh, make it stop,' she said, looking around wildly, convinced that the dream was really happening. And she was back in the kitchen of the farm. What was happening? Had she never left?

She shut her eyes tight and opened them again.

But everything looked the same.

And there was Callum, comforting John, crouched over the puppy.

'You can't keep them all,' he was saying.

'He's mine!' John had screamed. 'You said I could keep him.'

'No, I didn't. And what's that?'

There was a puddle of urine on the kitchen floor.

'It's a accident.' John stamped his feet, pummelling Callum with his fists. Callum caught them gently.

'I know. But we have to learn – have to work hard for stuff. Can't just have everything on a plate. When you're using the potty, then we can maybe look into getting a puppy.'

'I want Badger. Don't want another one.' John was inconsolable.

Frankie had rushed in. She swept John into her arms and cradled his ears in her hands. 'What are you saying?' she hissed to Callum. 'You can't take him away now. That's not fair.'

Callum shook his head. 'What good does that do him? Doesn't teach him anything.'

'He's three. He doesn't understand.' She crouched down to be on the same level as him and spoke in a loud whisper so that John wouldn't hear above his screams. 'Just leave him alone.'

'Fine, you deal with it, seeing as you're doing such a good job.' He reached over and grabbed John's arm so it was wrenched towards the floor, almost causing Frankie to topple over. She managed to hold on to him as he lurched – screaming – in her arms, very nearly hitting his head on the flagstones.

And then Callum shoved the little boy's hand in the urine.

'Feel that? You're going to have to get used to clearing a lot more of that up if you want a dog.'

*

Frankie heard a radio in the distance, and the sound transported her to another hospital, when Michael was just born, after she and the boys had been rescued from the van.

And she pushed her fingers into her ears to shut out the horrors of the world.

September 1998

When Frankie finally stepped out of the church, she was surprised by how bright and warm it still was.

She could hear music and laughter from the end of the road. And as she approached the taverna, a waiter appeared from nowhere. He swung open the tall wooden gate, welcoming her in like a sister, kissing her hand, and ushering her over to the far side of the restaurant. She felt her heart quicken. The courtyard was full. Long tables were lit up by candles and through the boughs of the cypress trees someone had stitched delicate strings of fairy lights.

She gazed in wonder, marvelling at the heavenly aromas of fresh bread mixed with lemons, roasted lamb and orange blossom and at the number of people – families – little children everywhere – couples – elderly men playing backgammon – all around her. 'Welcome,' the waiter said again with a smile and a flourish of the arm as he presented her table, laid out, along the whole length of the back wall, lined with stumpy cream candles wedged into old wine bottles.

'Only for one person?' he said, surprised, pulling out her seat.

One of the candles was leaning to one side and when the waiter turned away Frankie straightened it, checking it was stuck firm.

Vines clung overhead to trellises, and in the corner two young men were playing classical guitar. One of them was almost cartoonishly handsome in a hat and loose blue cotton shirt. He raised his hat to her with a smile as she sat down. She smiled back, quickly looking away and patting her hair to disguise the blush that she sincerely hoped would be concealed behind its prison of face powder. Something in his gesture reminded her of Omar and she felt a yearning.

She'd ring him as soon as she got back.

She felt suddenly a little self-conscious and very alone. She looked around her, realising that, unlike the other tavernas on the harbour, almost everyone except her was Greek, apart from one couple in the far corner who also looked British – or German maybe – older than her – in walking shoes and matching turquoise aertex tee-shirts – interrogating a waitress.

She felt a pang of guilt that the boys weren't with her, mixed with pride for having ventured so successfully off the beaten track. She kicked herself a little for having been so unadventurous every other evening.

After her meal she looked back over the notes she had made that week for the café idea. She had sketched a plot, in pencil, and drawn in some rough tables and chairs in the paddock. She'd allocate a patch of the garden, near the front, for the small restaurant-café for coastal walkers – more of a tea room, perhaps, if Bobbi had gone cold on the original chef partnership idea. And then the greenhouse for the nursery. She'd sell plants and vegetables all year round. It was bound to be busier in summer but she'd make it work, somehow. Other people did, didn't they? And the living area didn't need to be huge. There was only her, after all, now, wasn't there? So, provided the plot was big enough for the garden, she could get by with very little indoor space. It would be cosy. She couldn't wait to get back to start looking around villages. What was the worst that could happen?

Hadn't the worst already happened?

Several times, she thought, with a broad smile, accidentally catching the waiter's eye and flexing her ankle, noticing again that the ache had almost completely gone and trying to recall the very specific nature of the pain, annoyed with herself that she had forgotten so quickly what it had felt like.

She sat back, contented, and looked around at all the other people. She was so full and so tired that she thought she might actually fall asleep at the table, so – to the astonishment of the waiter, when he promptly delivered a baklava dessert 'on the house' – she graciously declined and ordered a coffee instead and the bill. He looked at her as if she had just slapped him in the face and shook his head, insisting, first, that she try the dessert. It was his wife's speciality, he explained, from Turkey.

And then he left her.

So, checking all around that she hadn't caused a scene, she dutifully tasted it. No-one was looking at her. It was warm and sticky and served with a spoonful of freshly made vanilla yoghurt scattered with pomegranate seeds. Frankie had never tasted anything sweeter. She hungrily ate a second and a third mouthful and scraped the plate with her spoon. And then she washed it down with the remnants of the ouzo.

As she started to gather her things together the waiter reappeared with the coffee. 'My wife says you would like some more baklava?'

'Oh, no, I couldn't possibly... I'll explode!'

He nodded rather seriously as he lay down the tiny cup of Greek coffee and a tumbler of water.

'That was all so delicious. Thank you. Please could I get the bill when you—'

He shook his head and turned to gesture towards a woman standing over by the wood oven. He shrugged his shoulders.

'My wife is coming now,' he said. 'She wants to know why you don't like her baklava.'

'Oh, no, I'm sorry,' Frankie started, checking her watch. 'It was delicious. I'm just so full!' She laughed and raised the cup to her lips. It burnt and her mouth filled with granules like drinking a bucket of wet sugared sand. She ran her tongue over her teeth and took a swig of water.

A woman sat down opposite her. 'My husband likes to joke,' she laughed, her eyes bright. She must have been about thirty, Frankie supposed, with dimples and shiny dark hair in a paisley red headscarf that she'd folded into a hair band. 'I know you like my baklava.' She pulled out a cigarette and tipped the candle towards herself to light it. Wax spilt on to the tabletop and she caught it between her fingertips and pressed it firm. 'Everyone in Crete loves my baklava.' She leant forwards and inhaled deeply. 'It's the best baklava in the whole of Greece,' she confided. 'Turkish,' she added in a whisper.

'Now...' She clamped the cigarette between her teeth. 'May I?' She reached for Frankie's cup and saucer. 'Nobody drinks coffee at night-time so I want to show you a little something special, okay?'

Frankie hesitated. It was getting late. Her taxi was coming at six the next morning and she wanted to get a good night's sleep. 'Okay,' she said.

'I'm going to read your coffee cup – your fortune.'

February 1979

After Michael was born Frankie left the hospital before being discharged, keen not to leave John any longer with Rosemary, the neighbour. Having hobbled from the bus stop to Rosemary's, the baby screaming all the way, Frankie looked up at the cottage and saw, with a pang of guilt, that John was sitting at the upstairs window. She wondered how long he had been there. She gave a little wave, attempting a smile, but as she waited on the doorstep, she could tell that he, too, had been crying.

She thanked Rosemary for her offer of a cup of tea but explained, above the screeching, with John tugging her arm, that she just wanted to get John home and try to settle the baby. She'd pop round the next day, perhaps, when they'd all got their bearings a little.

'So, has Baby got a name yet?' the old woman asked, peering into the pram, her voice raised to make herself heard above the piercing red scream.

'A what?' Frankie was suddenly bewildered. She heard a car pass and glanced over her shoulder at the rain, feeling a strong urge to run out into the road.

'A name, dear.'

She'd forgotten all about names. She and Callum had discussed a few but had never been able to decide on anything and now she couldn't think of a single one – her mind cloudy – like a blackboard wiped clean.

'Oh, silly me.' Frankie turned away so the old woman didn't

see her crying. 'No, not yet. Right, thank you, Rosemary. We'll see you tomorrow.'

'Oh, wait, dear. I almost forgot.' Rosemary turned. On the bottom stair was a small orange toy. 'Just a little something I found for Baby. I'm afraid I haven't wrapped it. I thought we had more time!'

'Oh, thank you.' Frankie stared down at the little orange knitted elephant, dressed in a pink paisley waistcoat. 'That's so kind.' She felt her face wobble. Not knowing what to say, she reached out clumsily and hugged the old woman, with one arm, around the shoulder, wiping her face with her sleeve as she did so.

That night, when she had finally managed to get John to sleep and while Callum was still outside locking up, she sat on the floor by the fire in her nightie, unable to stop the baby crying or to bear to pick him up again, her arms and breasts ached so.

She stared at the flames, her face as dry as a corpse, as if all the tears inside her had evaporated in the fire. She felt a deep hunger but had no energy left to make herself something to eat.

She stared at the little orange elephant at the end of the carrycot. One of the ears was bigger than the other. She couldn't bring herself to look at the baby's face. She felt he was judging her frown, spying on her, memorising each action to feed back to his father. She knew his eyes couldn't possibly see much beyond the edge of his cot at this stage and yet he looked at her as if to say, it's no use hiding from me; I've seen inside you, remember the dimensions of the hollowness there.

She reached over and turned the carrycot around so that he was looking towards the wall.

He screamed louder.

The Broken Line

She moved the bucket, where the nappies were soaking, closer to the fire – too exhausted to contemplate wringing them out.

The phone rang again. For the third time that day. She counted twenty-five rings this time, the noise reverberating in her head – through her teeth – as if she had bitten into metal. She knew it was probably Bobbi but she couldn't speak to her. She couldn't speak to anyone. All she wanted was silence and to be alone.

But still the baby screamed. There was no escape. He needed feeding again. And Callum would be back in a minute. Her breasts burnt and a sharp stab of pain flashed through her shoulders every time she moved. She wondered if there was anything left inside her to give.

She closed her eyes as if to pray, speaking the words out loud.

'I can't do this. I can't be the person I'm supposed to be.'

The baby fell silent at the sound of her voice. She barely registered it. And the tears started to fall again.

'I'm a nothing. I don't know what to do. I can't love this child. I hate it.' She kicked out at something and bashed her toe against the stone fireplace. She was weeping now. 'Don't make me.' Her breath heaved in ragged sobs and the heat was too strong for her eyes.

'I don't want it,' she hissed, getting up on her hands and knees and reaching for the tongs. 'Take it away.'

And then she said it again.

It was as if someone else were speaking the words, and she were merely the mouthpiece.

And then, without knowing what she was doing, she leant forwards and prodded the fire violently, shoving the burning log too hard towards the cot, so that it crashed from the grate on to the carpet.

She squeezed her eyes shut and clenched her fists to stop herself lurching forwards.

The baby let out a piercing scream.

'Frankie,' someone shouted. 'Get away!'

She jumped.

Someone shoved her, hard, to one side. She couldn't see him. A hand reached down for the cot.

It was Callum.

She stared, unable to move.

The log was lying, in full flame, in the hearth, just a few inches from the baby's carrycot. Glowing embers were stitched like jewels to the little orange toy elephant.

She crouched motionless in front of the flames. As if any movement of the air might fan the fire.

And without taking her eyes from the cot, as Callum held the little screaming child in his arms, she brought her hands together.

'I'm sorry,' she said. Over and over and over. She dropped the tongs in the grate.

She hauled herself up again, clutching the fabric of her nightie in one hand. She was shaking.

Although the baby was safe, she still snatched at the cot and dragged it away, tossing the toy elephant to the floor. Taking up the tongs again, she threw the log back on the fire, and grabbed a paperback from the bookshelf to crush the glowing embers on the carpet like a colony of ants.

And then she reached for the baby in Callum's arms, her mouth so dry that it hurt to swallow.

But he held out his hand and moved away from her.

The baby fell silent.

She watched the baby. His face was red. And he stared back at her in such a way that made her look away in shame. But

The Broken Line

not before registering the look in his eyes. For she knew, in that instant, from the way the light shone in his narrow grey eyes, that she would have to get away from that place. It didn't matter where she went.

But she had to get away quickly, she realised later as she sat in bed, beside Callum, in silence, forcing herself to bring the baby's face to her inflamed breast again to hide his eyes, wincing as she did so, noticing a trickle of blood on his chin as the little mouth clamped, hard, on her broken nipple, and squeezing her fingernails into the palm of her hand as she fended off the tears of agony. Because although she would never be able to pretend to be a proper mother to this child, she needed to get away before she did something for which there would be no forgiveness.

And she would have to, somehow, find a way to safely get rid of the child, to do the right thing, whatever she may – or may not – have wanted.

Because that is what the lines had said. That was her fate. They were there for everyone to see. That was her punishment. And she realised, looking down at the baby's cheek, too innocent, squashed into her aching flesh, that he still had no name. And she closed her eyes, knowing that the moment he had a name, she would be unable to pretend any longer that this child was not her son.

HIS FATHER'S SON

September 1998

'What do you mean, read my coffee cup?' Frankie frowned, glancing towards the gate. 'Like tea leaves? That sort of thing?'

'Exactly,' said the woman solemnly.

Frankie knew she shouldn't. And yet she felt a strange curiosity come over her as she watched the woman lay the coffee cup upside down on its saucer before lifting the cup off again, like a child hoping for a sandcastle, to reveal a little mound of granules on the saucer and a swirling brown trail on the inside of the cup. The woman moved the saucer to one side and placed the cup, with great care, between them. She sat in perfect concentration, only moving to inhale deeply on her cigarette.

Frankie stared at the saucer too, clenching her fingernails into her palm, willing her eyes to make sense – or pictures – of the meaningless patterns. And she wondered, a little uncomfortably, whether the woman really could read her future or whether it was some kind of joke that they played on gullible foreigners. But so what if it was? she reflected, leaning back in her seat. It was just a bit of fun, wasn't it? Completely different from that other time.

After a while the woman came to the end of her cigarette and flicked it behind her, still lit. 'I am not sure this was a good idea,' she said.

'What do you mean?' Frankie's heart quickened and she knew she should walk away. 'Can you see something?' She tried to laugh. 'Tell me. What is it?'

The woman was silent for a while. The expression on her face was grave and she did not meet Frankie's eyes. She traced a finger in the air above the saucer. 'It's not normally as clear as this – that's all. There's lots here. I can see a great feast – a banquet.' She indicated a shape – a fragile thread of brown, pointing and swooping. The longer Frankie stared at it, in the flicker of the candlelight, the more she convinced herself that she could see a table – a long twisting table – in miniature, as if from a fairy tale. 'And I see some sort of journey – a car – a boat or something,' the woman went on, hunched now over the saucer.

With one hand the woman absent-mindedly removed her hairband and folded the fabric neatly before putting it back and smoothing down her hair at the back. 'And now, just here,' she looked up at Frankie, catching her eye, 'in the middle of the feast, I see a big space.' She said the words slowly, making a smooth circular motion on the table with her finger.

Frankie swallowed and stared intently at the saucer.

'It's a departure,' she said. 'I've never seen one this pronounced. It is a great – how do you say...?' She looked up and Frankie felt sure that she saw fear in the woman's eyes. 'Danger,' she concluded.

'You mean I'm in danger? I fly home tomorrow. You mean the plane—'

But the woman was shaking her head. 'No. I see lots of people all sitting together. And a garden,' she said, pointing to two parallel lines.

'Oh, okay,' Frankie exhaled. 'That doesn't sound *so* awful...' She tried to laugh.

But when the woman looked up, her eyes had lost their shine and her mouth was downturned. When she spoke, it was as if she were looking into her own grave. 'Here,' she said, pointing directly in the centre, 'I see someone who has gone from your life.'

Frankie said nothing. Her heart had slowed down. And her face felt hot – the skin too tight – as if someone were pulling it taut.

'They will come back.'

'Who?' Frankie whispered. 'Is it my mother?'

But the woman shook her head. 'I can't see any more.'

'No.' Frankie grabbed hold of the woman's wrists. 'How dare you say those things to me?'

The woman stood up very slowly and took a couple of steps back.

Frankie was aware that people were watching. 'What gives you the right to say all that stuff? You don't know me. You know nothing about me. How do you think it makes people feel to listen to all that rubbish? Is it just a game to you?'

She needed a glass of water. She looked all around. Her vision was blurring. The music had stopped. She reached for the tumbler but the woman snatched it before her.

'You can choose what you see,' the woman said, staring at Frankie.

Then – just before splashing the water over the saucer so that it ran away from the table – she leant right into Frankie's face so that Frankie thought she was going to spit at her.

'But you can't choose what I see.'

And then she kissed Frankie on the cheek, retreating, with a firm goodbye, into the night.

Frankie was too stunned to speak.

She sat down, staring at the mound of dark brown sludge on the terracotta tiles beneath the table. The water crept towards her like a snake. She pulled her foot away and got up to sit at another table where, after a moment's hesitation, she promptly paid the bill and left, leaving no tip.

That night, when she finally fell asleep, her heart still racing from the coffee, she dreamt she was on an aeroplane. In freefall. All the oxygen masks had come down except hers, and although she was screaming for help the flight attendant kept bringing her trays of food, stacking them on top of one another, so she could no longer see above the seat in front as he explained to her, through his mask and snorkel, that she could not leave the aircraft until she finished her meal. And when the plane hit the sea, she sat upright in bed. It was four o'clock in the morning. She was drenched in sweat and her skin was still hot to the touch.

When she finally got back to John and Olivia's, it was late. She couldn't wait to tell them all about her holiday and hoped, desperately, that they were still up, as she fumbled with the lock, hauling her suitcase behind her.
But everything was in darkness.
She switched the hallway light on. 'Hello?' she called.
No-one answered.
They must already be asleep, she realised, a little disappointed, trying to decide whether to make a cup of tea or go straight to bed, as she glanced at her reflection, taken aback by how tanned she was. She checked the mail to see if anything had come for her, and wondered whether Bobbi and Al had received her postcard yet, and if it would suit them if she popped over to see them for a couple of days that week. She was hoping to look around a few properties in the St Davids area – for the café idea – and would massively welcome Bobbi's expert advice on the matter, not to mention any feedback on those menu ideas, if she had the time, that was?

February 1979

She didn't sleep that night. If the baby so much as stirred, she picked him up from his carrycot and fed him before he had a chance to cry out or disturb Callum, who slept soundly for the entire night.

In the morning, Callum rose early, checking she was feeling better, and promising to come back at lunchtime to give her a hand.

'We'll be up in Conway's until midday at the earliest,' he said, watching her uneasily. 'But I'll leave the van for you, just in case – in the old barn. I'll leave the keys in the ignition, you know, if there's an emergency or if you needed someone to come and get me, if you couldn't get there yourself, I mean.'

He lingered.

'But obviously keep the windows open. That lad's been fixing the exhaust but he needed a part so he's got to come back.'

Frankie didn't say anything.

Callum pulled the door closed behind him. The sound woke the baby. He immediately started screaming – a shrill wail – like the siren of an ambulance – that made her head jerk in time, as if someone were physically rattling her brain in its skull.

She picked him up and sat back down on the bed, holding him close to feed him dutifully, taking care to avoid his watchful gaze.

Afterwards, she changed him and waited for him to fall asleep before she lay him down in his carrycot. Then she grabbed a change of clothes for herself and for John and a bag of nappies and babygros and then she put on her winter coat, pulling the hood up so that John wouldn't see her crying if he woke up while she carried him, still fast asleep and wrapped in his duvet, out to the yard. She didn't know where she was taking him but she knew they had to get away.

The van was parked where it always was in the old barn. Methodically, she lay John down on the back seat and took off her coat to lay it over him on top of the duvet.

She walked blindly back into the house and fetched the baby in his carrycot, wrapped in his blankets and wearing the little white woollen hat from Bobbi.

Of course. She'd go to Bobbi's, she decided blankly.

She didn't need to think any further ahead than that.

She just needed to be somewhere else. She would stop and feed the baby on the way.

She rested him beside John before shutting the gate and walking all around the van to carefully close the windows.

Then she climbed in and started the ignition.

Music came pouring out.

She flinched.

It was far too loud – classical music – one of Callum's Poulenc tapes. She tried to turn it off but she accidentally knocked the volume knob so that a piercing high note screeched out, unbearable.

The baby woke up and let out a loud scream.

Although it was very cold and despite the violent shivering of her body, her skin felt too hot and the back of her neck was wet with sweat.

Her heart banged.

She looked up. There was a hole in the roof and she watched the snow falling down on them like feathers.

The exhaust fumes filled the van immediately.

She felt light-headed and afraid. Although she didn't know what she was doing, at the same time her mind had never felt clearer.

She switched on the heater and turned the fans up to full. She didn't fasten her seat belt. She didn't check the rear-view mirror.

She concentrated on getting rid of the music.

The baby's screams grew louder. 'There, there,' she said flatly. 'Don't cry.'

He cried even louder.

'It's okay,' she said, as if he could hear her. 'Mummy's here.'

Still he screamed. The noise made the bones in her ears vibrate. The smell of exhaust fumes didn't distract her and before long the fumes had completely filled the van.

She breathed in deeply, trying to ignore the screaming. There was a trace of petrol in the air, too. And she looked down to see a red jerry can in the footwell of the passenger seat. Although the smell made her nauseous, she tried to ignore the feelings in her stomach.

'It's okay,' she whispered again, her face stiff and cold. 'Don't cry.'

She rewound the cassette and switched the music back on, inhaling from the very pit of her being.

It started with just a piano and then slowly, as she began to feel a little sleepy, a second instrument arrived – a haunting woody sound that Frankie couldn't quite place.

The screams grew gradually softer, replaced in the end with a whimper.

And they lay there, united by the hot blast of air and the mournful melancholy of the music.

The melody crept higher and higher until she felt it no

longer belonged to the cassette but had moved inside her head and was trying instead to express something that she alone could feel. She felt her body start to fall into its arms. All was finally forgiven.

And then the baby gave a piercing shriek.

The music was suddenly much too loud.

He screamed and screamed and screamed. Frankie felt her heart lurch. The smell of petrol was overpowering. She clasped her fingers into her eye sockets until she couldn't see anything or hear anything.

And on he screamed.

But she could no longer hear it.

And then she became aware of a voice shouting. 'Get out. It's not safe. I haven't finished fixing it.'

It was that boy again, she realised abstractly, opening her eyes a crack – the boy who had driven her to hospital. But she knew, with a calm finality, that nothing mattered anymore.

Until a door was wrenched open and the car filled with light as Frankie registered, somewhere, that voice again, growing louder and louder. So that she couldn't tell if it was inside or outside her head as it boomed through the morning.

And a figure was standing over her, calling her name.

October 1998

Spa Shangri-La sat in an oasis of concrete just off the A34, approaching the Newbury bypass.

Susanna stopped the car abruptly in the entrance to the car park, lifting her spectacles to double-check the directions on her lap, to make sure they were in the right place.

'Isn't this lovely?' said Frankie, as if to herself, leaning forwards in the back of the car, fiddling with the clasp on her handbag and trying not to look at Olivia's expression through the wing mirror.

Susanna shot her daughter a long withering look.

Neither of them said anything.

After they had changed into their swimming things and put on the fluffy white robes that the girl on reception had provided, Susanna suggested they start in the main atrium.

Although no-one remarked on the décor as they padded in procession, like disillusioned ducks, the spa seemed to be undergoing something of an identity crisis, Frankie privately observed, suppressing a smile. It was part Himalayan retreat – with small grey stone Buddhas and strings of multi-coloured Nepalese prayer flags lining the walkways – and part Roman bath. The main pool in the atrium was decorated in miniature mosaic-inspired blue tiles, with a clumsily painted terracotta fresco on the main wall, showing a laurel-wreathed Roman emperor in profile – too orange and swathed in white robes – not unlike everyone else in the room, in fact, she reflected, selecting the lounger closest to the plunge pool. With the exception of some rather snazzy strappy sandals.

'Well, here we all are, then,' Susanna announced, tall and proud, dropping her robe flamboyantly on another lounger to reveal a navy and white nautical-themed swimsuit which sparkled in the low, amber light, with gold brocade straps and stiff foam cups to anchor her ample bosom. It gave her the air of having been upholstered – at great expense – in flammable acrylic-polyester-mix.

'Who's for a glass of fizz?'

Frankie felt underdressed by comparison in her trusty raspberry-print bikini that was so bleached now it was as if the Aegean sun had gobbled up all the fruit – even more so when Olivia casually revealed her immaculate physique – long flawless limbs shown off to perfection in a white strapless bikini and professionally applied hazelnut tan – the combination of which, especially with the addition of her smooth chignon and dissatisfied smile, made her look exactly like someone in that airline magazine.

As they stood there, examining the drinks menu, Frankie dived into the water.

The sauna was designed to look like a Scandinavian log cabin but felt rather more Swindon than Sweden, as Olivia had loudly remarked when they went in, already flushed from the champagne, and was nevertheless considerably hotter than either location. When Frankie sat down, the wooden bench scorched the backs of her thighs. There seemed to be no air in there at all and Frankie had to stop herself gasping when Susanna closed the door, too firmly, to prevent the people behind them from coming in.

'I wonder how the boys are getting on,' said Susanna, closing her eyes and loudly inhaling the hot dry air. 'I said to Brian, you mustn't be too pushy *vis à vis* cravats. It's John and Olivia's day. You must let them have the last say on the little touches.'

'Did you? Thank you.' Olivia breathed out loudly. 'John's really anti-cravats. I didn't want to upset Daddy, only I think John would feel way more comfortable with normal ties – you know – still something really special, obviously. He just says he doesn't want to feel like he's in fancy dress.'

Susanna snorted. 'It's a wedding, for Christ's sake, Olivia. It's not every day your only daughter ties the knot. Your father is paying for the bloody thing after all.' Eyes still closed, as if she were sunbathing, her face settled into a deep frown. 'Anyway, let's leave them to it.'

Frankie noticed the look on Olivia's face. 'I've no idea what I'm going to wear. I've seen a couple of things but nothing's quite right, somehow.' She turned to Susanna. 'Have you got your outfit sorted?'

'Yup.' Susanna pursed her lips. 'There's a little place in Henley. I always poke my nose in when we're at the regatta. It never disappoints. Found a gorgeous little shift – fuchsia – shantung silk – matching pashmina. Philippa Fennimore said it looked exactly like something she'd seen Princess Michael in.' She pulled a face. '*Vis à vis* hats – not so sure. I'm thinking: very classic. I found one that's nearly right. But it's cream. So that's obviously a no-no, unfortunately...' She shot Olivia a look. 'Probably have to start again. Brian won't like it. Nearly had an aneurysm when he saw the price tag on the pashmina. But I said to him, "It's not every day your only—"' She stopped, turning her face away. 'I said, "It's not up to you."'

No-one spoke.

The air was growing hotter and hotter.

After what felt like several minutes Frankie cleared her

throat. When she spoke, her voice came out too high. 'Have you and Brian been married long, Susanna?'

'Oh, far too long,' Susanna retorted. 'Coming up to twenty-seven years, can you believe? I said to Brian the other day, "Well, if we can make it through to thirty, then that's more than a good innings, isn't it?"' She laughed. 'Do you know what he said, the fool?'

Olivia shook her head unhappily but didn't reply.

'He said, "Well, I think I can probably get through the next six months – but I'm not sure about a whole year."'

Frankie gave a nervous laugh.

Susanna opened her eyes and looked Frankie up and down. Frankie sat up straighter. 'What about you? Will you be bringing a plus-one?'

'No, I don't think so,' said Frankie – her face so hot now she felt the blood might come bursting out of her eyeballs like in that gruesome film she'd seen on Channel 5.

Susanna's face scrunched into a smile that didn't meet the eyes. 'Brian's always saying, "What a pity Frankie's still single. Such a shame to be all alone at her age."'

'Oh, not at all,' said Frankie, bristling. 'I'm not alone – not at all single, actually.' She closed her eyes and breathed in deeply.

'Really?' Olivia elbowed her. 'Go on – spill.'

'Just a guy I've been seeing for a while.' She opened her eyes a crack to watch their reaction. 'He's an artist – a sculptor, actually – Egyptian – from Alexandria. Teaches at Oxford Brookes. It's all quite low-key. It's how we both like it.'

Susanna was staring at her open-mouthed but Frankie pretended not to notice.

After a while, Frankie turned to Olivia. 'You've been a great influence on John, you know. I hope he realises how lucky he is.'

Olivia looked surprised. 'Thank you,' she said with sincerity. She was quiet for a bit and then gave Frankie a smile. 'Thanks for booking everything today, by the way.' She leant closer so her mother couldn't hear. 'I actually prefer it when everything's not completely perfect.'

Frankie laughed. 'I'm so glad you said that.'

Susanna was watching them, a funny expression on her face. 'It's too hot now. The humidity settings are all wrong. Shall we swim?'

'In a minute,' Olivia said bravely. 'You go ahead. We'll join you.'

Susanna made no movement, as if she wasn't quite sure what to do next. 'Please yourself,' she said.

When Susanna had gone, Olivia turned to Frankie. 'I know this sounds weird but the first time I met John, when Mummy asked me what he was like, I said that he's one of those guys whose mum has done a really good job.'

Frankie stared at her, astonished, her face turning even pinker in the heat. She reached over and clumsily embraced Olivia. 'Thank you,' she whispered. 'That's such a nice thing to say.'

'He respects you, you know?'

'John?' Frankie raised her eyebrows. 'He has a funny way of showing it sometimes.' She laughed.

'You can tell. He's way kinder than most guys.'

Frankie didn't know what to say. But she felt she needed to say something. 'You're going to be great, you two. Marriage can be hard at times. Remember that. And please don't take any nonsense from John. He can be quite… challenging sometimes. There might be days when he'll drive you round the bend.'

Olivia smiled. 'Don't I know it.'

Frankie's mouth was dry and it was so hot now that her

heart was beating too fast. 'Shall we get out soon, do you think?' She stood up.

Olivia made no movement.

'I never had that closeness with my parents that John has with you.'

Frankie sat back down.

'Daddy can be quite hard work.'

Neither of them said anything for a while.

'He likes things to be just so – you know – everything's fine so long as it all looks good on the outside. But if you try and change the plan or disagree with him about anything – he can really go off on one.'

Frankie nodded.

'But it's not just that,' Olivia said quietly. 'The real issue that no-one ever bloody mentions is the small detail that he's been with someone else for years. Since I was seven, in fact. She was a friend of Mummy's.'

Frankie tried to think of something to say.

'He has times when he doesn't see her,' she said. 'Mummy knows; she's always known, although no-one ever says anything, do they?' She gave a mirthless laugh. 'Mummy pretends she doesn't care.' She shook her head. 'Whenever I ask her why she puts up with it, she just says, "Because he always comes back."'

'Right,' Frankie said, privately unsure why that would be seen as a positive.

'I don't think she'll ever admit to herself that she's terrified of being on her own,' Olivia said simply.

'It's not easy, being alone.'

'I suppose not. But something seems to have changed. Since John and I got together, I mean.' Olivia looked as though she was going to say something else and then stopped and glanced at the door.

Frankie waited for a while before speaking. 'That must have been incredibly hard for you, growing up with all that going on.'

'You *could* say.' Olivia laughed. She sat back and Frankie noticed her shoulders drop.

'If I tell you something,' Olivia turned to her; 'do you *promise* you won't tell John?'

'Of course.' Frankie laid a hand on her arm.

Olivia hesitated and looked down at herself. She sucked in her stomach and sat up straighter. 'Mummy was pregnant. I was going to have a brother. We talked about it all the time. I was seven. I remember it vividly. We had everything ready in the house. But then – a week before his due date – he died.' She snapped her fingers. 'Just like that.'

Frankie inhaled sharply, her hand rushing to her mouth. 'Oh, no. I'm so sorry. That's awful, Olivia.'

'She noticed the baby wasn't moving as much as normal. I remember her going into the hospital, so they could have a listen. Daddy picked me up from school that day. She was supposed to come home. And then she just didn't come home. And then my grandma came. But no-one told me what was going on.'

Frankie looked down, wrapping her arms around herself. Her face hurt.

'When she came home, two days later, she still looked fully pregnant, like the baby was inside still. But she told me that the baby had gone.

'I kept asking her, "Where? Why does it look as though it's still there, then?"'

Olivia paused as if she wasn't sure whether to go on. 'And Mummy and Grandma kept saying, "He's gone to heaven, Olivia."

'But at night when I'd gone to bed, I heard Daddy and Mummy shouting downstairs.'

She was silent for a while.

'And that was that. They haven't stopped since.'

Frankie tried to swallow but her throat ached.

'Mummy was different after all that. She stopped going out because everyone kept asking her if she'd had the baby yet and she couldn't talk about it. I had to get a lift to school with my cousin – you know George, the bridesmaid—'

'Georgina? Yes.'

'I think Daddy got together with this other woman during all that. I mean, wow, that's pretty low, isn't it, timing-wise? When you put it like that.'

Frankie frowned.

'He said Mummy was no fun anymore.'

Frankie felt herself stiffen all over.

'She used to stay with John and me – in the spare room, when they'd had a do. But I guess it's been a bit harder since you've been staying.' She stopped. 'Sorry, that came out wrong. I didn't mean—'

'No – I understand. I feel terrible. It must have been such a pain with me hanging around.'

'Oh, no.' Olivia brushed aside her concerns. 'Not at all. We love having you.' She looked away, deep in thought. 'I think John respects you for leaving his dad.'

'Does he?' Frankie stared at her in amazement, realising for the first time that she had no recollection of ever once discussing the subject with John.

'Anyway, cut a long story short: he had a daughter with her.'

Frankie stared, open-mouthed. 'Your dad? He's got another—'

'Yup. Zelda. Good name, right? She's fifteen now.'

Frankie shook her head. 'How did your mum cope with all of that?'

Olivia shrugged and looked into the middle distance. 'It's probably not connected at all. But Mummy and Daddy have been arguing more than usual lately and Mummy's started talking back. You know – standing up for herself. I think she admires you, too, deep down. Last night I heard her saying to Daddy, "Come on, then; when are you leaving us for good?"'

Afterwards, Susanna dropped Frankie at the flat and she and Olivia went back to Winchester so they could set off early the next day for the final dress fitting.

Frankie found John sitting alone at the kitchen table.

'You frightened the life out of me.' She switched on the lights. 'So, did you get the suits?' She stopped. 'John, what's the matter. Is everything okay?'

He wiped his eyes and shook his head. 'I can't do it, Mum.'

She sat down next to him and put her arm around his shoulder. 'What are you talking about? Come on, it's okay. What is it?'

'Just something stupid that Brian said. I don't think he even meant it like that. But it got me thinking. Liv deserves better. I can't be the sort of—'

'What's all this?' She faced him, placing her hands firmly on his shoulders. 'She's incredibly lucky to be marrying you.'

'I don't know,' he said softly. 'What if I can't afford the—'

She threw her hands up. 'Honestly, John. Please ignore that man. Brian Whitaker is a dickhead.'

'He's not *that* bad.'

'Yes, he is. He's what your dad would have called a little purple prick-cheese.'

'Mum!' John gasped.

'It's true,' she said grimly. 'And your dad, as you know, had *many* faults – too many to go into – but he was very astute when it came to people like that. All they care about is money. Money's just money. Sometimes it comes. Mostly it goes. But it's what's in here that counts.' She patted her chest. '*You* know that. So does Olivia.'

'I guess so.'

She leant back. 'Look, all families are tricky. And you're not marrying him, thank God. I wish you could have met your dad's dad.' She held her face in her hands. 'So controlling. So volatile. Textbook Scorpio. Made your dad look like Mother Teresa by comparison.'

But John didn't laugh.

He looked directly at her, his voice dropping. 'Why did you marry him?'

She took a sharp breath and looked down at her hands.

She started to speak but stopped herself. She suddenly saw Callum at the altar, waiting for her to arrive – the fear in his eyes as he scanned the faces of their families on the front pews. And then that moment when he looked up and saw her in the porch – that smile – before he turned back calmly to wait for her while everyone else turned to look – that seemed to say, you can go now; we'll take it from here.

And when she spoke her voice came out in a whisper. 'Because he always told it straight.' She sniffed. 'Like Michael, I suppose, in some ways. Never any frills with your dad.' She looked up at him and tried to smile, but when she saw John's expression, the muscles in her face refused to co-operate.

'I remember,' he said, looking away.

She reached for his hand. 'Hey—'

'I'm scared, Mum.' He wiped his eyes. 'I don't want to be like that.'

She shook her head. 'You're not like that. He wasn't kind, John, not like you boys.' She hugged him close until he started to pull away.

'It's hard work being married. But you're going to be great, okay? And you've got me. I'm always here if you need anything. And so's Michael.'

He pulled a face.

'He has his moments but he's got your back; you know that.'

'I know.'

She gave him a stern look. 'And promise you didn't give in to Daddy on the cravats?'

He laughed. 'What do *you* think?'

She squeezed him even tighter. And didn't let go this time. 'That's my boy.'

After he had gone to bed Frankie sat a while in the living room, thinking about everything that he had said.

She tried to picture John and Olivia a few years on, wondering whether they would have children, and whether she would prefer to be a Grandma or a Granny or maybe just plain-old Frankie.

And then she thought about Michael and wondered whether he would have children.

No – she thought, on balance, going up to bed, her mind turning back to that nice thing Olivia had said as she mentally rehearsed the wording John had scribbled down in preparation for her appointment with the bank, the following week, to talk about a loan for the café idea – or 'business venture' – as he had suggested. Probably not.

But that night she had the most vivid dream. She was back on the farm in the kitchen. Rain was hammering the windows and she could see Michael out in the yard – just a shapeless grey form trying to get in – a hole where the mouth should have been – failing – amidst the fury of the storm – to tell her something.

December 1998

The night before the wedding Michael had one of his dreams. He was in a garden but he knew it was the farm and he was trying to find his mum. He was both a young child again and a man, running away from his dad who was pointing a gun at him. Michael was wearing the white linen suit he had found in a charity shop on Broad Street the previous week. And as he pushed, knee-high, through a crowd of people, he realised everyone else was dressed in black, so that wherever he darted, his father found him, eyes trained down the barrel of his rifle. And Michael became aware that they were mourners, noticing – at the bottom of the garden – a row of granite gravestones.

But then, just as he lurched to the ground, his father was there, looming above him. Everyone was screaming.

'Stop!' Michael tried to shout but no sound came out. And then, just as he realised he was going to die, his father turned away, pointed the gun into his own face, and pulled the trigger.

There was an explosion of silence.

Michael sat up, his sleeping bag soaked with sweat. He could hear Monira downstairs on the telephone, and when he opened the window, he caught the clattering, wheeling sound of geese flying over the house.

He knew, however pointless it might be, that he had to at least try – one last time – with his dad.

He wondered what time it was.

Aware of a gnawing hunger, he quickly pulled on the white suit – his mind flashing back to the dream – and brushed his teeth. His mouth still tasted bitter. He went downstairs and made himself drink some water and have a slice of toast but everything tasted sour.

He looked around for some shoe polish before wiping his boots with a damp cloth.

If he left now, he could just about get to Misselden and still get down to Southampton by two, in time for the wedding.

He knew he should really phone ahead, but Monira was still chatting and he didn't want to interrupt so he decided he'd just call in on his dad. He gave Monira a little wave and mouthed goodbye as he went.

He hadn't seen him for months.

He drove quickly, reaching the farm just after nine.

He felt a flutter in his stomach as he parked the van on the grassy verge. His mouth still tasted funny.

The gate was closed, almost entirely concealed by the wild rose that was so overgrown now that, as Michael wrestled with the heavy rope on the latch, a thorny bough caught his sleeve like a child tugging on its mother's arm, begging her to come back.

His father's car was not in the drive and the stable doors were closed.

It struck Michael that maybe his father wasn't there. But where else would he be at this time on a Saturday morning?

He hesitated before climbing over the gate, looking down at his suit, already creased from the car. Why hadn't it crossed his mind that his father might not be there?

He still had that strange thirst and he was properly hungry now, too.

Gem the sheepdog was lying in the middle of the courtyard.

'Gem!' He whistled, expecting her to pounce.

She made no movement.

He stopped, sensing immediately from the way she was lying that something wasn't right. He tried to ask himself, doubtfully, whether perhaps she was simply asleep.

But she was too still – fully exposed – making it impossible for any life to still be there.

He stood over the corpse of the dog. It looked smaller – lighter than Gem had been – as if diminished by her absence, lying on its side in a little patch of dark brown blood, its six teats and tiny sharp incisors exposed – the head perfectly preserved – like a stuffed dog mounted in an antiques shop.

Michael looked all around him. There was no-one there.

He hesitated as he approached the main farmhouse. The curtains were open a crack and he peered in through the living room. It looked untidier than normal, with plates and empty bottles on the table and a chair upturned in the middle of the room. And then he saw a flicker and realised that the television was on.

He went around the side and knocked on the door, pulling back the lavender as he tried the handle.

Inside, the kitchen stank of cigarette smoke. Michael gagged and left the door open.

There was mess everywhere – scrunched-up paper all over the floor; books; CD cases; clothes; plastic bags.

A bottle of scotch was lying on its side, with no lid on, on top of the piano. When Michael picked it up, he saw that it had spilt on to the sheet music propped up on the stand below, where his dad had been playing. It was the faded yellow collection of Chopin's nocturnes that his dad had taught him to play. His face felt heavy as he looked around for a cloth. And as he wiped the sticky ivory keys they rattled, out of tune; the higher notes had stopped singing altogether.

He covered his mouth with his sleeve.

He went into the corridor. The door to the gun cabinet was open. He started to breathe more quickly, his eyes darting around the room.

He heard a shuffling noise from the living room.

'Who's there?' a voice bellowed right behind him.

Michael jumped.

His father quickly dropped the gun.

'Dad.' Michael stepped back, his eyes fixed on the rifle hanging from his father's hand. He caught his breath. 'Put that away,' he shouted. 'You nearly gave me a heart attack.'

His father looked very thin – frightened, too, and had it not been for the fact that he was dressed – uncharacteristically smartly, in black suit trousers and a shirt – Michael would have been excused for thinking he had roused his father from a dream. His eyes and face were red and puffy; his hair, overgrown and matted. A sparse beard did little to hide his despair, making his face look gaunt – at once very young and very old.

Michael sighed slowly and reached out and touched his dad on the shoulder. 'Are you okay?' He frowned. 'We need to put the gun back.' He tried to lead him to the cabinet but his father held on to it defensively.

'It's fine,' his father said, retreating to the sofa and laying the gun down where he'd been sitting. 'What are you doing here anyway? What time is it?'

'It's nine – half nine.' Michael watched the gun out of the corner of his eye. 'What happened to Gem?'

His father looked away. 'I had to put her down, didn't I? Poor sod.' He turned to Michael. 'Where've you been? What's got into your mum? Who's that *man* hanging around her? And why's she taking all that money out? I can't believe she's fucking me over – *still* – after all these years.'

Michael stared evenly at him. 'I think you need to let it lie, Dad. I'm not sure if you know but it's John's wedding today, so—'

'What the blazes do you think I'm dressed up like this for? Morris dancing? I'm going down after I—'

'I'm not sure that's a good idea.' Michael reached out to steady his father. His shirt felt damp and smelt sour – of stale alcohol and smoke.

His dad pulled away.

Michael looked out the window at the courtyard. Two crows were jumping around the carcass of the dog. 'What was wrong with Gem?'

He grunted. 'Last of the cows have gone.'

Michael looked at him, confused. 'I thought the test came back inconclusive?'

'Doesn't matter. Got to get rid of the lot of them. Big con – whole thing.' He looked around. 'Sheep are next. We're ruined. Completely unsustainable. Everyone's told them.'

'So what are you—'

'Can't bring it back from this, Mike. They've got no idea. Civil servants – just kids – bleating some rubbish off a bit of paper. Do you know what he said to me? Get this: "Have you *considered* adapting your agricultural strategy, Mr Webb?" Well, I came this close, Mike…' He raised his fist. 'Never set foot on a farm. No idea how these things work – the generations of work – expertise – the *family* tied up in it all. Gone.' He clicked his fingers.

Michael didn't know what to say. He looked all around him. The smell was making him queasy. His cheeks tingled and his stomach felt hollow.

'I half-thought about sitting him down, explaining it. Not a single day off in twenty-five fucking years. I even thought about looking into it – you know – going to court and all. And then I just…' He stopped and looked at Michael as if he had forgotten what he was talking about.

Michael steered his father to a chair.

There wasn't much in the fridge: a few eggs, a giant Tupperware tub of butter and a jug of milk that was crusted, yellow, around the rim. Michael prised open the drawer of the freezer where he was surprised to find half a bag of white sliced bread amidst the empty ice-cube trays that rolled back and forth on a bed of loose peas like ball bearings.

'I'll do some eggs,' he called out uncertainly as his father went into the other room.

All the pans were dirty so Michael pulled up his sleeves and cautiously approached the sink. It was full of dirty plates and glasses and the stench punched him in the nostrils. He reached for the plug but there was something slimy blocking the plughole. He gagged and snatched his hand away. His mouth filled with saliva. It was pale yellow vomit. It couldn't be anything else. He hurriedly turned the hot tap on, and rinsed the stuff off his hands, looking all around for some washing-up liquid.

Holding his breath and turning his face away, he forced the handle of a spoon into the plughole to try to dislodge the chunks as he concentrated on trying not to be sick himself.

After they had eaten, Michael's father was calmer and explained to him that he wanted to show him something important in the main barn.

He went into the other room and came back with a piece of paper. 'I've been sorting a few things out lately,' he said, sitting down heavily to pull on his boots. They looked odd over the suit – and too big – as if they belonged to someone else.

'It's mainly about this place,' he went on, gesturing to the mess that encroached from every angle. 'The rest of it's long gone but this place – and the Willows – we can hang on to these. Should get a good price. It's too much for one old sod on his own anyway. More trouble than it's worth, especially with your mum walking out on us and John getting married and all…'

'Right…' Michael nodded cautiously, wondering again whether John was aware that their father knew about the wedding.

'And I was thinking that you might take it – if you want it, that is.'

Michael didn't know what to say.

His dad left the piece of paper on one side and grabbed a bunch of keys on his way out as he headed off towards the stables without a glance at the dead dog.

Michael followed. 'But where will you—'

'I won't be here.' His father stared straight ahead, his voice flat.

Michael felt an unfamiliar pain spreading across his scalp and down the back of his neck. 'Why not?'

His father went into the stables and came out with a big metal spade. 'I'm going away for a bit,' he said, heading back to the dog.

He bent down and wedged the spade underneath the dog's stomach to lever it like a dead mouse that a cat had brought in. The dog's head and legs hung heavily on either side as his father staggered towards the barn. 'Thought I'd best get some things sorted first.' He lay the animal down in front of the iron gate of the barn.

Michael couldn't look away from the dog's eyes, half open still, as if she were keeping watch even now.

His dad drew back the thick metal bolts.

The noise must have disturbed the pigeons roosting in the eaves, for when he started to pull the gate across, Michael heard flapping as the birds flew off in all directions, like bats.

His father waved one of the birds away with his hand and picked up the dog again on the spade.

Michael held back. 'I can see you've got a lot on. I'm going to head off now.'

His father turned to face him. The look in his eyes was one that Michael didn't recognise. He stared right through him. The metallic grey of the irises looked suddenly very small, exposed and afraid amidst all the surrounding red. He seemed shrunken, too, crumpled up, and his arms shook under the weight of the dog. When he spoke, his voice wobbled. 'Why are you here anyway? How did you know?' His voice broke and he hung his head, his shoulders juddering as the dog slid off the spade, landing like a bag of cement in front of him.

He fell to his knees.

'I don't know.' Michael stretched his arms around his father's shoulders and rested his cheek on his dad's back, holding him there.

His father was openly sobbing now. His whole body heaved and he let out a strange low wail. 'I needed her.'

Michael closed his eyes, his jaw clenched, the angry tears soaking, hot, through his father's shirt.

'I knew she wouldn't come. But I...' His father was struggling to get the words out. He shook his head. 'I didn't want to be alone.'

'It's okay,' Michael whispered. 'You're not alone.'

'I thought the *only* person who might come is old Mike.' He gave a squeaking laugh. 'But I never really believed you'd be here, Mike. Not after what I did – landing you in all that mess with the police.'

Michael didn't say anything. Across the yard he watched a pigeon pecking at something on the ground. From nowhere, an image flashed through his head, of his mother, lying in a hospital bed.

He stiffened and pulled away.

'I never thanked you, Mike. Never said sorry – not to anyone.'

Michael nodded, feeling a pull in his heart.

'I'm sorry about your dog, too, when you were a kid.'

Michael hesitated. 'That was John, Dad.'

'Was it?'

'It would mean a lot to him – I know it would – if you said sorry to him.' Michael reached out reluctantly to embrace him again.

Neither of them spoke, their ragged breathing slowing with every intake, and falling, eventually, into a deep, synchronised calm.

Michael felt him sit up a bit and although he loosened his hold he waited before letting go entirely.

His father sniffed and seemed to come to his senses. He looked up.

It had started to rain.

'And then, when I realised no-one was going to come, I decided to do something I've never done before.'

Michael felt unease starting to curl its way around him again.

'I prayed.' His dad laughed out loud and marched up to one of the pens.

Michael breathed out, long and hard.

He watched his dad crouch down and embrace one of the sheep. It had black markings on its face and it was perfectly still in Michael's father's arms, watching him.

'You must think I've lost my marbles.' He retrieved the dead dog and carried it to the same pen, laying it down in front of the animals. 'I think she'd want to be here.' He nodded at the sheep. 'Sailors at sea and all that.'

Michael swallowed. He nodded slowly and stepped backwards. 'And do you think God heard you, Dad?'

'What? Look, it's time you got going. Go and get that bit of paper. It's all there. There's a copy with the solicitors as well. But don't breathe a word to your mother.'

Michael hesitated. He knew it was dangerous to ask but he knew it was more dangerous not to. 'What about the gun, Dad? I don't think it's safe to—'

His father turned on him. 'Who d'you think you are, preaching at me?' He pushed Michael in the chest, causing him to stumble. 'You've no business coming here,' his father muttered as he walked back across the courtyard and into the house, leaving the gate of the barn open. 'Now get out of here before I change my mind.'

Michael headed back to the van, tussling again with the gate before turning to raise his hand, just in case his father could see.

He stopped, surprised to see his father, standing there in front of the house, so small now, and slumped, wearing his heavy shoulders as one would an old overcoat. And Michael was taken aback to feel a rush of pity for the man – his face crumpled in anguish, like an abandoned child.

Michael held out his arms. 'It's okay, Dad. God will never desert you. You can always—'

But his father suddenly lurched forwards like a wild animal, skidding on the gravel, disturbing a cloud of dust so that Michael almost didn't see what was happening in the very moment that his father raised the gun.

He pointed it straight at Michael.

'Dad—' Michael cowered, his arms in front of him, like a shield.

And then he felt an almighty force smash him in the chest as he was hurled backwards against the wooden gate.

And throughout the courtyard there resonated a tremendous, thunderous flapping of wings – like applause through a cathedral – as a huddle of pigeons and doves exploded, in a flash of white, scattering soft grey-brown feathers that rained down on the barn from the heavens.

December 1998

That December had been unusually mild and it rained incessantly in the days leading up to the wedding. Olivia had meticulously planned every detail of the day, plotted out clearly in rotas that she had taped up in the kitchen in the summer.

Although she did her best to conceal her discomfort, Frankie was finding the atmosphere in the flat suffocating, especially combined with the endless discussion of the seating plan. But she wasn't able to move in yet to that endearingly wonky little cottage that she had found when she went to stay with Bobbi and Al for the weekend, not long after she got back from Crete.

It was in a hamlet just a few minutes' drive from their house, overlooking Cardigan Bay. And it turned out that Bobbi knew the owner, who agreed, when he found out she was Bobbi's sister, to let Frankie try it out as a rental for a few months, before she made up her mind whether or not to buy. But that meant waiting until January. So, Frankie had nowhere else to go in the meantime, with the exception of the occasional weekend in Oxford with Omar.

John and Olivia had been so hospitable to her since the fire and she hated to be ungrateful but she felt so apprehensive and irritable, for some reason, whenever she pictured the wedding that she wondered whether she would be able to cope in that flat until the new year.

She hadn't been sleeping well, and kept waking from horribly vivid dreams of being trapped in a burning building. There was no-one, apart from Omar, of course, and Dr Carmichael, in whom she could confide regarding her anxiety about the wedding day or her fears that Michael had been the one responsible for the fire.

She obviously didn't dare say anything to John.

Not that John would have even cared, it seemed to Frankie. Usually so astute in these matters, he seemed oblivious to everything but Olivia these days. And although she understood why Olivia felt uneasy, it irritated her that John didn't appear to notice the marked shift in Olivia's mood when her parents came to stay, dismissing her fussing as endearing, holding up his hands as if to say, 'don't look at me, Mum – that's Liv's department.' When Olivia decided, two days before the wedding, that she had changed her mind on cake decorations, Frankie felt ready to leave the country.

Despite only living a short drive away, Brian and Susanna had decided to come to stay for a few days beforehand – mainly to help out – but also so that the infamous cousins, of which there seemed to be about twenty-five, as far as Frankie could gather, could have the run of the house in Winchester.

'I mean, for God's sake, as I said to Brian, what's the point of having all that bloody space if you can't put people up when your only daughter ties the knot?'

And so Frankie had inexplicably found herself offering to sleep on the sofa to let the Whitakers have the spare room, which she had regretted the moment the words left her mouth.

They arrived armed with acres of folded lace and proceeded to sit on that same sofa for the best part of forty-eight hours, forensically debating the depression approaching from the west, while Frankie served them meals. They never once acknowledged her help. Frankie half-hoped the warm front would wash the wretched table plan clean away – and the wedding guests to boot.

John wasn't much better, hypnotised by Olivia's prettily scrunched-up nose as she agonised over whether to ditch the lavender bags altogether for the favours – and just go with something more conventionally Christmassy. And Frankie found herself questioning, as she hid in the kitchen one evening behind a large glass of red wine to help her face the second run-through of Brian's speech, whether perhaps it was just the wedding itself rather than the letter she'd sent to her mother, or the prospect of Michael turning up that was making her feel so anxious.

Of course Michael knew he had been invited, originally, to the wedding. And John had definitely sent him a save the date card to that house in Reading – as had Frankie – but he had never officially replied.

And Frankie was not the only one unsettled by his silence.

Olivia had made it quite clear the night before, when they were printing out the revised seating plan, that she didn't think it was at all appropriate anymore for Michael to be there and she'd feel better if John gave him a quick call to double-check that he wasn't coming.

'What if he just turns up, out of the blue? Or thinks he's still the best man or something? Weddings are stressful enough, trying to please everyone,' she had pointed out, accidentally waving the scissors dangerously close to John's face. 'The last thing I need is some huge family hoo-ha right in the middle of everything else we've got to get done.'

'Is that Michael?' Brian had called from the kitchen.

John rolled his eyes. 'He's my brother, Liv.'

'Come on, John. When's the last time he called you or came to see us or did anything for us, in fact? I've only met him once.

And I'm sorry but it's incredibly rude to not even reply. I don't see why I should invite people I hardly know to my own wedding. There. I've said it.' She slung the scissors across the coffee table, stepped back and crossed her arms. 'Whoever they are.'

Frankie could see John's jaw was clenched and he was staring at the floor.

'I don't think there's anything to worry about,' she said. 'I'm sure Michael won't come – what with all he's been going through. He's not been in touch for a long time...'

John frowned at her and shook his head in irritation.

Susanna poked her head around the door. She brought the cotton reel to her mouth and snapped the thread between her teeth like dental floss. 'Is everything alright, Olivia?' She re-threaded her needle. 'Is this Michael we're talking about again?'

Frankie ignored her. 'But I agree with John,' she said. 'It's only right. I'm sure he won't turn up but, I'll tell you what, why don't I just make a little card for him, just to be on the safe side, like the one for John's grandmother.' Sweeping aside the sprigs of holly that she'd been trimming, she grabbed the pen out of John's hand. 'They probably won't come, but if they do, we can just pop them on the table at the back.'

Susanna flopped into the sofa. She glanced around with a dissatisfied frown. 'Well, I'm not at all convinced we need to invite him,' she said, squinting at a corner of the lace that she was sewing. 'Brian,' she hollered. 'Did I leave my glass in there?'

Frankie's face stung but she spoke evenly. 'Michael is John's brother – and my son, let's remember. And if he does – by some miracle – decide to make an appearance, then we will all make him very welcome. Won't we?' She smiled sweetly.

Susanna raised one eyebrow and shot Olivia a look, before returning to her sewing.

December 1998

On the morning of the wedding itself, for the first time in months, Olivia was nowhere to be seen – presumably immersed in a sepia foam of bergamot champagne, thought Frankie meanly, trying again not to think about her own disastrous choice of bridegroom and picturing herself back then – so joyful and young and stupid – in all that glorious shimmering silk.

The silence was perfect and Frankie would have been tempted to spend the day in bed – had there been a bed in which to hide – and had she not been lying awake all night instead, with her face squashed against the spine of the leather sofa in the middle of the living room.

But she dutifully dragged herself to the bathroom to quickly shower and get ready before the Whitakers emerged, pulling on her long-sleeved olive-green dress with the wide neck that suited her narrow frame and reminded her, once again, of that lovely going-away dress she had worn on her honeymoon.

She frowned and wiped off most of the lipstick.

Then she fastened her necklace – a chunky gold chain that had been a gift from Omar. It sat, cold, against her slender throat and she smiled in spite of herself, relieved that her hair hadn't flattened overnight. The lighter colour was better, she noted, and the layers made it look thicker and heavier than before. Her hair looked almost golden, in fact, in the early morning light that fell diagonally from the Velux window. And when she stood on the toilet seat to try to see the maroon shoes with a chocolate brown ankle strap that she had bought especially, even though they were too expensive and too high, she was unsettled to confront, side-on in the mirror, the reflection of a woman at least ten years her junior.

She hesitated before clambering down and unbuckling the shoes. She'd wear the flats.

And then, staring herself straight in the eye, she put them back on, before reapplying the lipstick, thicker than before, and left the hat on the back of the door.

When Frankie went into the kitchen for breakfast, she was astonished to find an envelope addressed to her, on the kitchen table, in Michael's inimitable script.

'John,' she called out. 'Did you put this here?'

But there was no reply. He must have gone down to the marquee already to help set up.

She sat down and opened it, taken aback by the alarming familiarity of Michael's handwriting – minuscule and all over the place – and she could see him crouched, writing it, immediately – hear his voice, clear and confident as she read the words, as if he were sitting right beside her, still in his school uniform, the Bible in his hands, guiding her to the right passage.

Dear Frances,

Frankie couldn't help but smile.

I need you to understand that I never meant to hurt anyone. I took the gun because I was afraid of what Dad might do. He has always known that.

She felt something pulling inside her, as if to test the workings of the heart.

I am still worried about him. I tried to talk to you about it once before but it wasn't the right time. And I will never forgive myself for what happened next.

Please be careful.

Frankie stopped reading.

She thought she could smell smoke. Grey speckles swarmed in her peripheral vision. She closed her eyes and swallowed hard, trying not to think about anything.

But the memory would not go away – of Callum – late one night, at the farm. It was after Christmas; Michael was almost one. It had taken her ages to get the boys to sleep and when she came downstairs Callum was sitting in the dark – his back to her – at the piano. The only light came from the twinkling bulbs of the Christmas tree. The piano was closed and the tumbler of whisky rested precariously on the sloping walnut lid.

'If you ever walk out on me again,' he'd said, sliding his empty glass along the smooth surface of the wood, so that they both watched it smash, in slow motion, to the floor, 'do you know what I'll do?'

The noise instantly woke Michael again so that he screamed out loud.

'What did you do that for?' she snapped at him, switching on the light and looking around for the dustpan and brush. She marched upstairs and picked Michael up, carrying him back down with her before the noise woke John.

But when she came back into the kitchen, Callum spun round. He was pointing a shotgun directly at her.

Gripping Michael with all her strength, she had hurled herself to the floor, feeling his body tighten in her arms; he made no sound.

'I'll go up there and I'll shoot the boy in his bed.'

John was awake now. And screaming.

'And then I'll come back down here and I'll shoot that little bastard, too. And do you know what? I'll say it was an accident – that the boy was playing with it.'

She tried to read on but all the muscles in her face were pulled taut and there was a pain creeping across her scalp.

'When I was a child, I spoke as a child, I understood as a child, I thought as a child, but when I became a man, I put away childish things. For now we see through a glass darkly, but then face to face. Now I know in part, but then shall I know even as also I am known.'

Thank you for everything.

Love never ends.

Michael.

Frankie looked out of the window. One of the bridesmaids – Olivia's cousin, Georgina – was carrying trays of canapes out to the car, dressed in a leather biker jacket and Susanna's navy wellies – her hair blow-dried, in giant rolling curls.

Her mouth was too dry.

She knew she should phone Michael. But she felt as if all the air had been knocked out of her and as if it would require too much energy even to stand.

She forced herself to get up, dialled his number and waited, clutching the receiver so hard, as it rang on and on, imagining the sound of his voice, that her ear ached from the pressure. But she didn't let go until the line went dead.

Although Frankie managed to pull herself together, dry her face and regain some semblance of composure, she couldn't get the letter out of her mind.

John stopped her, on the way out to the car, and took her to one side. 'Are you alright, Mum? You look really pale.'

She didn't know what to say but she nodded, holding back the tears. She buried her face in his jacket and inhaled deeply. He smelt of oranges and cinnamon. 'I love you, John. Don't mind me. I'm just nervous. Good luck today.'

And she prayed, all the way to the hotel, that Michael would come.

But Michael did not come.

And although she tried not to be angry with him, she felt she was going to explode if she couldn't see him, couldn't hold him close, couldn't tell him how wrong she had been or how much she adored him.

When two o'clock had been and gone and the bride and groom were saying their vows in the gazebo, under giant baubles of mistletoe, she realised Michael definitely wasn't coming and that she should really just try and focus, for once, on her other child.

John's eyes were glistening and the look on Olivia's face – only partly visible from the way she was standing, as if for a magazine shoot, with one foot pointing to the guests, hair tunnelling down her back and landing, as if by accident, at the deep V of the cream cap-sleeved gown – was one of pure unexaggerated delight, her warm smile unspoiled by the clouds gathering just above the photographer's head.

Perhaps Michael had just decided not to come.

To his own brother's wedding.

Despite being the best man.

She tried to see the funny side – to make light of it, inside – but her heart was too heavy.

After the ceremony, Frankie walked over to the marquee, the cold grass snapping and tugging at the heels of her new shoes, as if to pull her under the ground. She wished, again, that she had been brave enough to bring Omar after all. She'd wanted him there initially, but had grown uncomfortable with the idea as the date grew nearer, feeling it would be better to introduce him to the boys on a less momentous day – maybe in the new year, or so – after the dust had settled. And so they'd decided to meet the day after instead, in Oxford – perhaps go for a walk around Christ Church Meadow or a glass of mulled wine in the Turf garden if they'd got the heaters up; or do something nice, at least, just the two of them.

She looked around at the couples, shivering, pretending to chat to one another on the lawn as they glanced over their shoulders for the sight of a familiar face. Two little sisters crouched, giggling, at their mum's ankles; she was talking to someone, nodding earnestly, one hand behind her back to patiently remove flakes of soggy confetti they were stuffing in the waistband of her skirt. And in the distance, Frankie caught a glimpse of Bobbi – all in black – just a flash of red lipstick – talking to their dad, with Al beside her, chatting to an elderly woman in a navy tailored coat.

'Who's that?' Frankie muttered.

And although she couldn't see the woman's face, for a moment she allowed herself to hope.

But just then, someone stepped in front of the woman, blocking Frankie's view so that she had to stand on tiptoes to be able to see around them.

She stared.

There was something in the woman's posture – slightly stooped – as if the thoughts weighed too heavy for those narrow shoulders – that told Frankie it must be her.

She had come.

After all these years of wanting.

And she felt completely – and strangely – blank.

She wondered why she didn't feel more surprised. More emotional. More anything, in fact. Instead, all she felt was a stillness.

As if things were simply as they were – a picture put back

on an empty wall. Not especially good, necessarily – nor bad. But true, at least, and in the right place.

And just at that moment, her mother looked over, saw Frankie watching her, and stumbled, stepping back slightly. She gave a nervous smile and raised a hand.

And suddenly Frankie saw that she looked younger – like looking into her own reflection.

And they were as one again – the before and the now – all the intervening years collapsed in on themselves like a fan of cards.

And Frankie waved back.

She knew she should go over. And she would. But afterwards – after the ceremony, the speeches and everything. It was too much right now. They needed proper time.

And then someone tapped her on the shoulder and she jumped to find a huge smiling circle of John and Olivia's school friends. And after chatting for a few minutes to John's best man, Dominic, Frankie excused herself, pretending she needed to check something with the table decorations, before hurrying away, acutely aware that her mother was the only other person there who had come alone.

The marquee was empty and she sat down – by the heater – on the long bench that lined the back wall to form the top table, like a very cold, secular reconstruction of *The Last Supper*, she had observed to herself, reflecting again on the last-minute changes to the seating plan and wondering whether that made her Judas – and Susanna, presumably, just the Messiah.

Consulting the laminated table plan at the main entrance to see where her mum would be sitting – next to Michael – she snatched his name card from the small overspill table at the back of the marquee and shoved it – pretending to adjust the candlesticks – between her and Susanna.

As people started to filter in, she surveyed the clusters of meticulously positioned guests, tucking into bread baskets, in silent joviality, at pristine round tables. They seemed oblivious to the tiny lace lavender bags that were almost obscured by the butter dishes now and the wreaths of holly and ivy that had taken Frankie two days to arrange.

The sprigs of berries were too small, she noticed later, as she listened to Brian's speech for the fifth time that week – shouting to make himself heard above the sound of the hail that thundered on the canvas, like a herd of water buffalo.

Frankie wished she'd brought a warmer jacket. She could feel a draught behind her, and the occasional spatter of rain that crept, jerkily, between her shoulder blades and down her back. She did not dare turn around but sat motionless as if on stage while in her mind she imagined the gap in the canvas growing bigger and bigger, with the rain blowing through, picturing it collecting in little wrinkled pools on the black hessian flooring before it swept open to engulf the lot of them.

Every so often the microphone made a high-pitched screech and Brian winced theatrically, crouching down, his hand – still clutching the list of his daughter's achievements – pressed against his left ear, like an old-fashioned radio deejay with the sound turned up too loud.

John was smiling broadly, his arm soldered around his bride's corseted waist while she wiped her eyes on Susanna's late mother's blue antique handkerchief as Brian turned from his daughter's dressage rosettes to her extensive academic triumphs.

Frankie saw something out of the corner of her eye.

She jumped.

A figure was slouched in the doorway at the side of the marquee, hands in pockets.

Michael.

No.

She gasped.

It was Callum.

Of course it was Callum. There was no way he would have ever decided to stay away.

All the blood rushed to her face and her knees trembled, concealed by the tablecloth. She could almost feel the heat from the fire again – smell the smoke.

She clasped her hands together and gripped her knees, looking down at the table as if she hadn't seen him, so thin as to be almost unrecognisable, in a black suit that looked funereal against the dull grey of his shirt. His face was stubbly and his hair dishevelled over an open-necked collar.

He was staring straight at her.

She was trying so hard not to look at him that her eyes throbbed. But all she could see was his face that night in the kitchen, at the piano.

How dare he ruin everything for all these years?

Frankie tucked her hair behind her ear. Her jaw was so tight she felt the tendons might snap.

She sensed a movement and glanced up as Callum shrugged a shoulder in acknowledgement before looking away to survey the room.

Although she didn't look directly at him, she was intensely aware of his outline.

Well, that was that. She wasn't going to let him ruin John's wedding day. She looked around for her mum; she could see her listening carefully to the speech, a smile on her face. Frankie couldn't bear for Callum to somehow find her mum or say anything to her before she'd had a chance to speak to her herself.

She followed Callum's gaze and then she caught a glimpse of Michael. She breathed a huge sigh of relief and felt her whole heart lift. He was standing at the back of the crowd, all in white. He raised a hand to her.

She beckoned Michael up to the top table, patting the space beside her.

And then he slipped from view.

She stared at the space where he had been. And a few seconds later she saw him again, heading up the aisle, at the side of the marquee, and round the back of the top table.

He sat down beside her.

She gave him a big smile. 'I love you,' she mouthed, feeling safe at last. Everything was as it should be. He'd come back. And her mum was finally there. She had to pinch herself. How on earth had it all worked out like that?

Everything was going to be alright from now on.

She leant towards Michael. 'I'll be back in a minute,' she whispered.

Trying not to distract too much attention from the speeches, she slipped around the back of the table and out through the flap into the catering tent.

And then she marched right out of the marquee into the rain.

'Callum,' she shouted. He was still leaning against the doorway watching the speeches.

He turned, surprised. 'Hello, Frankie.' He looked her up and down. 'Looking very flash. Likes the slutty look, your new fella?'

She could feel her whole body shaking. 'You've got a nerve showing up here. I'd like you to leave now, please.'

He looked through her.

'If you don't,' she went on, crossing her arms in front of her, 'I'm going to call the police and have you removed. Immediately.'

'There's no need,' he said.

He looked years older than last time she'd seen him, his arms and legs thin, where the muscle had wasted.

'They're already looking for me.'

'The police?' She stood up straighter. 'Why? Because of the fire? I know it was you.'

He frowned. 'No, not that. Because of Michael.'

'What's Michael got to do with anything? He's only just arrived. I've told you to leave the boys alone.'

'Who's just arrived?'

'Michael. He's right there.' She turned and pointed at the table.

She stared for a moment – the light bouncing from the glasses – the swirling movement of the guests. It reminded her of something.

For there, next to Susanna, in the space where Frankie should have been, was an absence.

'Frankie,' Callum snapped his fingers.

She jumped, forgetting, in that instant, that he was still there.

'Michael's gone.'

'What are you talking about?' she said, glancing automatically over her shoulder to see if she could see him.

'He's dead. He died this morning.'

She recoiled. 'How dare you?' She pushed him, hard, in the chest so that he stumbled backwards. 'To think you can come here and say all this shit to me? On today of all days.'

His eyes were all shrivelled, too deep in their sockets and she noticed he was shivering. When he spoke, it was in a whisper, almost as if he doubted what he was saying was true. 'I shot him, myself.'

Her whole body shuddered. She stepped backwards. 'There must be something very wrong with you.'

But she was surprised to realise, as she stared at him, that although she was shaking, it was no longer because she was afraid.

'I feel sorry for you, more than anything. I really do.' Her voice shook. She reached out and patted him awkwardly on the shoulder, like a child. 'But I'm telling you now: it's time to go.'

And then she turned around and walked straight up the central aisle of the marquee to the top table.

December 1998

Frankie sat down, dutifully raising a glass to the bridesmaids, and looked over to John who was waiting for the cheering to die down.

'And now to absent friends,' John went on, 'including my own little brother, Michael, the artist formerly known as Best Man – who sadly couldn't make it today.' He turned to Dominic, laying a hand solemnly on his shoulder. 'And so a double thank you to Dom, here, for those kind-ish words about me just now. As you all now know, Dom and I have been friends since we were seven. And throughout all those years at my side, he's been a truly outstanding Second Best Man.'

There was a ripple of laughter but only Callum continued to whoop.

Frankie deliberately avoided Callum's gaze but she saw John look over – his face tightening – when he heard his dad's voice. John looked down, busying himself with his notes, and he tapped the microphone as if to check it was still working. She could see his hand was shaking.

'It's okay,' Frankie called to John as quietly as she could, leaning right across Susanna so that the other woman cried out in annoyance, pushing her chair back. 'I've spoken to him. Ignore him.'

John nodded and raised his glass to Callum. 'And to Dad… speaking of absent friends,' he added, almost inaudibly. Frankie watched her mother turn in curiosity, with the rest of her table, to inspect the rather louche-looking character now leaning too heavily against the delicate lace awning that had been pinned, with such care, by the mother of the bride.

As Frankie sat there, still as a corpse, she imagined it buckling, in slow motion, under Callum's weight and realised she had been holding her breath.

'Hear, hear,' Callum called out in response.

Frankie glanced briefly at him, noticing that he was not smiling, and she felt that old acidic sting at the back of her throat as her heartbeat gained pace.

Why had he said all that stuff? She scanned the crowd. People were whispering. Where was Michael? She focused intently on refilling her water glass.

Ignoring the sound of someone standing up to one side of her, she tried desperately to concentrate, for once, on her eldest son but her eyes were drawn, as if by an external force, continuously back to her husband.

Something brushed her shoulder. She jumped as if she had been electrocuted. 'Michael! There you are!' She felt such an extreme rush of warmth coursing through her that she thought she might fall backwards off her chair, as a pale willowy figure, all in white, sat down beside her, a solemn expression on his face. She reached for his hand just as he moved away.

She couldn't stop smiling. 'Thank God you're here,' she whispered, her hand in front of her face. 'I love you.' Tears of relief fell freely. 'I'm so proud of you.'

As she sat there, in front of all those people, she realised she didn't care anymore what they thought. She just had to tell him how much he meant to her. She had wasted almost twenty years not saying it – never saying anything she needed to say. Always saying those silly little things that anyone could say – that didn't even need saying in the first place.

He reached over and mouthed something to John who ignored him.

As she twisted to listen to John, she surreptitiously glanced at her mum and back to Michael. Despite his pallor, his skin was unblemished – his hair short and neat, as it had been the last time she'd seen him. He'd obviously recently had it cut. And she felt an overwhelming sense of peace, like being bathed, under a ferocious sun, in a stream of the coolest, clearest water.

As John finished speaking, people stood up to clap and cheer and someone raised a toast to the happy couple.

Michael stayed seated, leaning forwards, his chin resting on his hands that were clasped together as if at prayer.

He turned to her as if he were about to say something, and then he was gone.

'Michael?' She spun around. 'What…?' She looked over at her mother. And then to Callum. But Callum wasn't there either. 'Where's Michael?' she hissed.

And then something – or some*one* – shoved into her – sending her lurching to one side as a champagne flute toppled, crashing down on to a plate – fragments of glass descending, like sparkling snowflakes, across the tablecloth.

And then he was there again.

But not fully there – just a glimpse like a reflection caught on an uneven surface.

He looked like a child again.

Susanna was brushing the broken glass on to a plate with a napkin while people continued to cheer, oblivious. Frankie caught sight of Olivia's laughing eyes – bright with tears. She was whispering something to John.

People were getting up, starting to mill around, and she noticed a little huddle of waitresses waiting in the wings, preparing to bring out huge silver platters of profiterole mountains and pavlovas.

There was a commotion at one of the tables. Her mother

was standing up, staring straight at Frankie – a look of concern on her face. She reached out a hand.

Someone was tapping her on the shoulder. She jerked away. It was John, reaching across the place where Michael had been. He was asking her something but there was a ringing in her ears and she couldn't hear him.

And then she became aware of someone speaking. Although she knew it was Michael she couldn't tell if the voice was real or inside her head. It was as if he were calling through a tunnel. She hid her face in her arms.

'Love never ends.'

She felt a hand press, heavy, on her head. Another on her shoulder. Warmth seeped from her scalp down her neck and through her body.

And then, looking up through the crowd, she saw it – a sudden movement.

Callum pushed forwards. He was holding something in front of him.

He raised his arm and pointed the sawn-off shotgun directly at her.

'John!' she screamed, jumping to her feet and lurching to one side as she flung her body in front of him. 'The gun!' She dragged him – plates smashing – to the floor.

A cry rang out – like that of a wild dog. And then the air filled with noise. Even before it came. Frankie felt it more than heard it – as if the ground had shifted beneath her and risen up to smash her in the face. And then came the sound – like a massive explosion – that she realised, only in that instant, she had been both dreading – and expecting – for all those years.

The gunshot.

And everything dissolved.

December 1998

What felt like hours later, the world reverted to chaos.

Tables were overturned and people ran in a screaming stampede from the marquee.

'Michael!' Frankie tried to shout. 'John!' She looked all around for her sons, but she couldn't make a sound.

Someone was shrieking above her – the noise, up close, intolerable. She crouched under the table, amidst stamping feet, broken glass, jagged shards of china and – everywhere – the unbearable stench of lavender.

She squeezed her head between her hands to block it all out.

Someone lurched over her and was pressing her neck with their finger. She couldn't breathe – couldn't tell whether she'd been hit.

There was blood everywhere.

'Michael!' she tried again.

He was nowhere.

'John!' she tried to call, looking down at her motionless limbs – a mesh of ripped flesh, broken glass and blood. 'Michael's dead.'

Was it her own blood? she wondered dimly, trying to scan the air for the boys.

It was Susanna. It must have hit Susanna. She had fallen back off the bench and was clutching her arm – blood, sprayed like red ink, across her pink pashmina; her hat had fallen over her face.

And then John appeared, his body too large and swaying

as he towered over Frankie, shouting. 'John,' Frankie wanted to cry out, feeling all the air come rushing out of her body. She tried to holler again as he turned away from her, his face in his hands. 'Where's Michael?' she wanted to say.

Susanna's eyes were open too wide as her hands convulsed.

Someone else was hurt, too, and a little huddle had formed just to one side of Susanna. It must be Brian, Frankie told herself wildly.

Olivia, who had immediately taken charge, was directing individual faces, within the blurred horde of screaming onlookers, to call an ambulance, while Brian stood over Susanna.

John was standing, howling, above her, like a child once more, his mouth wrenched in a black hole, his arms – blood-spotted – pumping up and down, while a voice in the darkness shouted for a doctor.

And then she saw a glimpse of Bobbi; no – was it her mother? They were both there – faces overlapping now, features merged.

Frankie knew she should get up and help but she couldn't seem to focus or to get her legs and arms to work properly. She couldn't see Callum either. And so she stayed exactly where she was. She closed her eyes, in case he could still see her, as if she had known what was coming next – that it was what he had been waiting for all those years.

And then the proof – the second shot.

Before the silence that told her that Callum was gone – that it was over.

She tried to sit up but her body was no longer connected to her mind.

John was slumped on the floor beside her. He was moaning and he had his back to her, cradling a body in his arms.

Frankie felt as if she were underwater and yet she realised, as if seeing herself from a great height, that the body that John was holding was her own. She saw her foot – her own foot – the shoe missing. And the algae green of the dress, bleeding, now, into a mesh of red, like a body lost at sea.

She heard someone, from a great distance, emit a strange animal wail.

And then she saw Michael again.

Lying on the floor.

'Michael!' She reached blindly for her son.

Although his face was unblemished, his bright white suit was soaked in blood. And as she stared at his face, forcing her eyes to work harder than they had ever worked, she realised that she couldn't be certain it was him.

And she became aware of a great searing pain in her scalp as if her brain were physically pushing against her – denying that this man's body could ever truly be her son.

And then, just as suddenly, his body vanished.

'Michael…' Her vision turned grainy and her stomach dropped as her eyes roved, searching for him.

She snatched the edge of the tablecloth, pulling down a cascade of plates and glass.

Someone was speaking to John.

A woman – a paramedic.

It was too loud, right next to Frankie's face.

'It's the bride's mother-in-law,' she heard the paramedic say. 'She's been shot, so I'm going to have to ask you to move, sir, if you don't mind. I know you've had a terrible shock.'

Strong arms reached down and lifted Frankie, under the armpits, from the floor. But she couldn't focus properly.

She looked at John, unable to comprehend what was happening.

John was shaking his head. 'Mum!' he cried, pushing the paramedic out of the way and pulling at her body, trying to heave it closer to his face but it was too heavy so that her head rolled to one side as John collapsed on her broken chest.

And then something was shoved over her face so that everything went dark as Frankie became aware that, although she felt as though she was still there, it was perfectly clear to everyone else that she had been dead for some time.

December 1998

The police waited until around half-past eleven the following morning before they knocked on the door of the spare room. John had been in there all night, sitting on the floor, and Frankie had been with him, keeping him company. The officer wanted to inform John that they had found what they believed to be his brother Michael's body the previous afternoon, on the farm.

'No!' John leapt to his feet, backing away towards the wall as though to get away from this world. His face was so contorted now it was as if the pain had burst through his skin to physically rearrange the individual components of his face – leaving just a weak, estranged impression of the man he had once been – no more substantial than a reflection in a carnival mirror.

The sound of his wail – like a dying hyena – filled the building.

'It was following a report,' the officer went on, glancing at the paper in his hand – unsure how to proceed – 'of the sound of a disturbance from a neighbouring property.'

'It's not true!' John shouted, hurling himself to his knees and burying his face in the bed covers.

The officer waited, head bowed, for several minutes.

And then he started to talk again, raising his voice to make himself heard above John's screams of fury.

'He appears to have died from a number of shotgun wounds to the chest. I'm terribly sorry, Mr Webb, I know this must be very difficult for you after everything you've—'

'Go away! Leave me the fuck alone.'

The officer nodded. 'We'll be off as soon as we've finished here, Mr Webb. I'm so sorry to be delivering such tragic news.' He wiped away the sweat from beneath his shirt collar. 'We believe it happened yesterday morning, about ten, eleven o'clock or so. And it appears, at this very early stage of investigations, that your late father was responsible for that attack, too.'

John was shaking his head like a lion devouring a lamb.

'Leave me alone. Stop talking.' He reared up and lurched towards the officer, fist raised as if to swipe at him.

The officer cowered, his hands shooting up to his face.

Frankie reached out and seized John's wrist.

'What—' John flinched; his arm sprang back. He stared at the empty air.

The officer stepped backwards and stood in the doorway. When he spoke again his voice shook and his eyes were filled with tears. 'But I must inform you that we will be needing you, as soon as you feel strong enough, that is, to come down with us to the morgue to help us identify your brother's body.'

John let out a strange guttural moan that sounded not quite human.

He crouched back down by the bed, staring up at the officer – his eyes blank and shrunken by the agony, like holes where the rotten flesh has been dug out – as if he didn't understand the words the officer was speaking anymore.

And then everything fell silent.

'I can't hear anything,' John said, his voice detached and unfamiliar. 'I need you to go away now.'

'Of course, of course, sir,' said the officer, raising a hand and glancing over his shoulder as he retreated very gently from the room.

*

Frankie sat with John for the remainder of the day, leaning against the bed, with her arm wrapped around his shoulder, wishing she could take the pain away from him.

She knew it made no difference. John couldn't hear her, but still she tried to soothe his tears. 'It's okay, John. Don't cry. I'm here.'

And just before the police left, at around six o'clock in the evening, the same officer knocked tentatively on the door.

Frankie could hear the clang of saucepans from the kitchen and pictured Bobbi helping Olivia prepare dinner.

'So sorry to disturb you again,' he said nervously, trying to hand something to John. His hand was shaking. But John – head buried in his knees – didn't even look up. Frankie wasn't sure he was even aware that there was anyone else there.

'We found a little card at the farm for a Frances, you see. It'd fallen out of your brother's pocket. The duty officer thought it was a girlfriend or a wife or something, but then your missus explained...' He paused. 'We wasn't looking for a mother.'

As if that made it better, somehow, that her child was dead.

But there was nothing left to say.

So, the officer bent down and left the card on the floor at John's feet.

And eventually, the next day, when John felt ready to join the others, Frankie read it.

It was a Christmas card, she realised, handmade. She looked at the picture – a square, painted a rough grey, with a drawing inside made from a single unbroken line – suggesting a woman holding a baby.

She opened it. In miniature capital letters, in pencil, as if written by a child, were two words: THANK YOU.

And as she stared at the formless wash of the woman's background she felt sure she could see wings emerge from the grey before withdrawing to the air, like finding a momentary meaning in a cloud.

Frankie stayed in the flat for some time, keeping vigil.

No-one noticed her.

She felt bad about leaving John but she knew it would do him good to go for that walk that Olivia had suggested, with Brian and her mother and Bobbi, after they'd been to see Susanna in hospital – just to get some fresh air and have a change of scene.

And it would do her, Frankie, no end of good to get out of the house. She'd go mad if she just sat there crying all day. Michael wouldn't want that. He'd want her to at least do something useful, wouldn't he?

And then it hit her again – like a punch in the stomach – the realisation that he was gone.

She looked down at her hands, clasping them together, her flesh numb.

The temperature dropped that night and it snowed for the remainder of the week.

It was a privilege to be able to spend time with John and Olivia, witnessing the way they held each other together, speaking their truths, doing their best to sort the chaos into some form of order, dealing with the endless calls from the police, the coroner, the solicitor and the funeral directors. And to start to get the farmhouse and Willows Cottage ready to put on the market.

She helped wherever possible.

Willows Cottage needed a complete clear-out. There were

boxes full of all sorts of junk and piles of old furniture that hadn't been touched since Rosemary had died. The old woman had even left her knitting bag, Frankie realised, having a little go herself one evening, discovering with surprise, as she looped the orange yarn over the stubby grey plastic needles, that she still remembered how to do it, deciding after a few rows to make a little something – a toy for a child – a mouse or an elephant or something.

And Frankie found that it made her feel better – as if the activity itself were helping to physically block out the thoughts and the pictures of Michael that crowded into her head like a swarm of ants the minute her hands stopped moving.

The sun woke her one morning, some weeks later – at the end of January, it must have been, on the day of the funerals, she realised – and she was relieved to find that although the wind blew colder than ever, the snow had finally stopped.

John and Olivia would still be asleep; it was too early to pop by, so she thought she'd go for a little walk around the farm.

Frankie's feet were stiff in her shoes, and as she fumbled with the door keys, the metal pressed so cold into her rough hands that it stung and she contemplated going back inside for her gloves.

She walked carefully, for although the gritters had got rid of any trace of snow on the main roads, the lane was still snow-lined on both sides, leaving only a narrow glassy aisle.

The sky was a strange pinkish-grey like the feathers of a dove. It seemed to brighten as she walked. And the scene was at once peculiar and yet immediately familiar.

As she approached the farmhouse, she saw that the Sold sign had finally been taken down. There was a van parked in the outhouse next to the stable, a pair of feet sticking out from underneath the exhaust pipe as sweet clarinet music poured from the radio.

The front door of the house was wide open. And inside she could hear voices.

She looked up, noticing the way the light reflected off the upstairs window, bathing the whole scene in an inky wash of pink.

And then the windows were flung open and a young woman leant out. She was crying. 'Is anyone down there?' she called out. 'Where *is* everyone today?'

Frankie tried to call up to her but the young woman couldn't hear her and she stepped away from the window, back into the darkness of the room.

Frankie went inside.

The woman was kneeling against the bed – sobbing – head in hands. The duvet cover and blankets were strewn all over the place and a small suitcase for the hospital – half-packed – lay open beside her.

Frankie reached out and touched the young woman on the shoulder.

The woman flinched and stopped crying. She looked all around her as if she had heard something. And then she turned to the space where Frankie was standing and she looked right at Frankie, holding her gaze – keeping it there – like a promise.

'Hello?' the young woman said, her surprise momentarily stopping the tears. 'Is someone there?'

'Don't cry,' Frankie said. 'Everything's going to be alright.'

The woman said nothing but stayed very still. And then she held her stomach with both hands. 'It's starting,' she said, her voice flat and her face twisted. She let out a sob, her jaw clenched. 'I can't do this anymore.' She punched the mattress.

Frankie held her. 'Don't be afraid,' she said, over and over, until the woman's pain had begun to subside. 'You'll love this child.'

She stayed there with her as the hours passed and the morning lightened, watching the lines of worry start to fade from the woman's face as she allowed herself to be soothed, as if a wave had washed over her.

And all that time the young woman talked to herself. 'You can do this. You're nearly there now. He'll be gone all day. This is your chance. You *can* love this child. You *can* start again. Just do it.'

And as the pains grew stronger, something else in the young woman seemed to strengthen until she was unable to breathe from the pain. And then, when it had passed, she hunted around for the phone and dialled quickly, looking out the window and scanning the yard.

'Bobbi? It's me.' She breathed out in relief.

From the window, Frankie watched the young woman and her child stagger across the courtyard, trawling the heavy brown pram behind them. And as they closed the gate, the young woman turned back to the house and looked up at the window. She raised a hand to Frankie and smiled, as the little boy chattered on alongside her as if there had been no lull.

Aeroplanes had been flying and as Frankie watched the morning sun start to seep like spilt orange juice through the cloud, she saw they had left intersecting trails, forming a gigantic cross on its side as if the sun had been shouldering its weight until now but the time had come to hand it over.

And all at once, through her mind, as if this were the moment she had been waiting for, ran the words of Michael's prayer.

Love never ends. For we know in part and we prophesy in part, but when the perfect comes, the partial will pass away.

And without knowing where she was or what she was

doing Frankie became aware that everything was changed and she saw something – or someone – who had no form – coming towards her. And as she fell to her knees, she found herself speaking the words out loud. 'Love never ends.' And she was seized in an all-encompassing embrace – suddenly lifted from this earth by an almighty force.

And she knew it.

And it was the beginning.

And it was the end.

***

Pulling the gate closed behind them, the young woman bent down to hug her son.

'Now remember what we said. Auntie Bobbi's on her way and she'll pick you up from Rosemary's. So, you be a good boy for Rosemary until she gets here and then Mummy will see you at Bobbi and Al's house, okay?'

He didn't say anything.

After a while he looked up at her. 'Will Daddy be there too?'

She frowned and glanced over her shoulder. 'No. Daddy's staying here.'

John nodded. 'What do you think the new baby will be called?'

'I'm not sure.' Frankie stood up and squeezed his hand as the pain started to come again. 'What do *you* think it'll be called?'

'I don't know. Maybe he's called John, too?'

'Oh, I don't think so.' She smiled down at him. 'Because *you're* John and you're the most important person in our family so we can only have one John, can't we? The new baby will have to have a different name.'

'Maybe Michael then?' said John. 'Like the boy who's mending Daddy's van.'

'Yes,' she said, surprised. 'Maybe Michael. Why not?'

He thought about it for a while as they set off towards the cottage. 'I don't think there's enough space for Michael.' He turned away with a sniff. 'Michael can stay with Daddy.'

She stopped, leaning forwards, resting her hands on her knees, as she waited for the pain to subside. When it had gone, she hugged him hard. 'We're going to love him, John. More than the world. We're going to be a team.'

And in that instant, she sensed something – behind her – in the courtyard.

She turned back to the house, uncertain whether she had remembered to lock the front door.

She looked up at the window – the light catching on the glass. It dazzled her for a moment. And although she wasn't sure at first what it was that she was looking at, she could see something – a shape – framed in the window.

She squinted to try to distinguish the edges of the darkness from the form that suggested a figure – a woman. It looked like her mother, the way the shoulders sloped – gazing at the sunrise.

And without knowing why, Frankie raised a hand in acknowledgement.

For the longer she stared, the more she could see, as the clouds shifted to reveal one side of the woman's face – each detail lit up as if engraved in metal – all the lines of all the families converging in that one expression of what can only be described as rapture, as she saw, at last, how the darkness had illuminated the light.

ACKNOWLEDGEMENTS

It has taken several years to write this book and many people have helped me. I would like to thank: Mark Lucas and Peter Straus for encouraging me to take my writing seriously; Jon Wood, my phenomenal agent, for having faith in me and for his supersonic ability to pinpoint exactly what works and what doesn't; and Juliet Mabey, Shadi Doostdar, Jenny Parrott, Polly Hatfield and the team at Oneworld for their enthusiasm and panache, helping to turn a story into a novel.

Thank you to my fabulous friends and family; my wonderful parents and sisters for your boundless love and support all my life; and to my beloved children and Will, for your patience, love, unbeatable company – for absolutely everything.